Making Contact

uses of language in psychotherapy

Making Contact

uses of language in psychotherapy

Leston Havens

Harvard University Press
Cambridge, Massachusetts, and London, England

Library of Congress Cataloging-in-Publication Data

Havens, Leston L.
  Making contact.

  Bibliography: p.
  Includes index.
  1. Psychotherapist and patient.   2. Psychotherapy—
Language.   3. Psychotherapy.   I. Title.
RC480.8.H38 1986   616.89'14   85-24912
ISBN 0-674-54315-7 (cloth) (alk. paper)
ISBN 0-674-54316-5 (paper)

Preface

Today we have an abundance of therapeutic devices to alleviate psychopathological symptoms. But more and more people are seeking help for less dramatic (and more stubborn) difficulties, those of character and situation. Many patients are hidden from us, not showing who they are or what they want for themselves. The frankest arrive saying, "My life has no meaning" or "My life isn't going anywhere" or "I only go through the motions." Then there are those with no life to express: not only are they purposeless, but there seems no one present who is able to have a goal or vision. Still others gain what presence they have from the invasion, manipulation, or imitation of outsiders. A few of these are outright imposters, consciously taking up the roles of others. More often such patients find they have assumed an existence merely because it is available or fashionable, not because it is their own. These difficulties can be situational as well. For example, the person is controlled by a spouse or an employer; she or he only follows "orders." The orders may come from outside or, in addition, from dominating figures long since internalized. An observer wonders whether the new tyrants are selected, created, or imagined. And sometimes the individual does not know he is a slave.

I will discuss these infirmities under the categories of absence and isolation, of domination and submission. The goals sought in therapy are to "find the other," to confirm and develop a presence, to manage social forces impinging from inside and outside, sometimes to create and often to resolve conflict. Implicit is a view of being human or human Being, that is, a normative ideal or goal of psychic health, which I will characterize as the capacity to be alone with another, personal freedom or self-possession, and liberation from the need either to invade or to be invaded. In this way, psychotherapy introduces to personal experience what the concept of democracy introduces to political experience: opposition to tyranny. Although rights of free speech and assembly are patently protected, with us still are the forms of inner and interpersonal control: destructiveness and surrender. A society in which psychological isolation and domination prevail makes being human a rare and hazardous venture.

The same point can be made from the perspective of evolution. The struggle for existence originally meant survival of offspring, passing on the genes. Existence also has a psychological meaning, as we learn poignantly when we see physical life continuing without the conditions necessary to sustain the inner sense of being alive. Just as medicine became a powerful tool for the preservation of physical life against those species and adaptational defects inimical to humans, so do psychiatry and psychology now battle for our species' human existence.

The evolutionary analogy illuminates how the contributions of the various psychiatric schools can be usefully integrated. Biological and descriptive psychiatry identifies those threats to existence that are responsive to drug therapy. Psychoanalysis looks at the difficulties in development that make a full existence precarious: the need for balancing the powerful forces struggling inside the individual, the inevitable costs to human individuality of the equally necessary adaptation to the social and physical world, and the complex and still evolving nature of human procreation, childrearing, and family life. The part of psychoanalysis that relates failures in development to failures in social environment, so-called object-relations theory, also has a separate status as social or interpersonal psychiatry. The development of this environmental viewpoint has greatly widened psychiatric understanding and allowed access to new kinds of cases. Unfortunately, it has aggravated professional sectarianism as well, which the evolutionary analogy again illuminates. Medicine defends against a host of parasitic species. The most successful of these defenses, still necessary because of the continuing evolution of species, has been against bacteria. The findings of social psychiatry clearly indicate, however, that humans are parasitic on one another. As a consequence, psychiatry exposes and opposes the actions of many members of its own species.

The problem is not new to medicine, in the area of public health at least. Here it has long been obvious that many of the greatest dangers to man arise from other men, and not only through ignorance or carelessness. It is no accident that concern about nuclear weapons emerges so strongly in the public-health community, or that the most original figure in social psychiatry, Harry Stack Sullivan, was among the first to speak of the nuclear danger.

Formidable difficulties arise for psychiatry from the fact that pathogenetic human beings exist. This intensifies opposition between the psychiatric schools; for example, family therapists accuse psychopharmacologists of quashing the symptomatic protests that can be useful in civilizing family life. Or the generations are set against one another, as young people blame elders for their own inadequacies. Homosexuals dislike heterosexuals for homophobia, which makes a viable homosexual existence almost impossible. Men strive against women. The list can go on and on—in fact, social analysis reveals any group as at least a partial oppressor of some other group. None of these protests can be casually dismissed because oppression is real. So psychiatry and psychology must judge these complaints and, as part of that judgment, begin to define the conditions necessary for freedom and self-possession.

It is no coincidence that existential psychiatry should emerge at this time. The growing awareness of the psychological dimension, of the precariousness of human existence, and of the competing and often oppressive demands on human life makes the existential search for human Being and human beings seem, once again, the response of the organism to the demands of its world. This effort can be thought of as a psychological speciation in which members of the human race are separated into those who are fully human and those who are not.

Here is a partial response to the failure of biological and descriptive psychiatry to give an account of the human background of disease. Without such an account, there is no way to judge the extent and dangers of any pathological process. Also, existential psychiatry has trespassed upon psychoanalysis, most notably in the work of D. W. Winnicott and Heinz Kohut, who have developed what Freud only touched on: the place of ideals, values, authenticity, and selfhood in human sickness and health.

Suppose a species were to conquer the world, only to discover that its greatest danger is not the emergence of new species, but itself. What if it realizes that, in order to survive, it has to modify old predatory habits that served very well before? Perhaps this species would signal its fresh resolve by allowing malformed children to live and the physically unfit to grow and multiply. Would not that be the first clear evidence of a new "psychological species," which puts human existence before the physical? Human existence would then have one simple definition: it would be whatever maximizes the fullest survival of the human species. Now, if continued predation threatens not only whomever is preyed upon but the whole species in this age of genocide, and if all forms of slavery are incompatible with human existence, then outer limits have already been set on the definition of human Being. Giving someone freedom does not mean the freedom to invade. Instead, the test of freedom is the capacity to be present without either disappearing or invading. The new psychological species would be able to manage the invader without becoming invasive itself. An ideal of mutual respect supplants the former goal of predation, and for the same purpose: survival.

The psychotherapeutic means I offer in this book are directed against absence, isolation, submission, and domination. They are a means by which human presence is discovered and defined, and a weapon in the constant struggle for existence.

A word about my organization and terminology: The book would seem to be arranged chronologically, moving from establishing empathy with the patient to coping with the world outside to creating viable personal goals. It should be understood that any such chronology is artificial, for the sake of pedagogical convenience, if you will; the course of real therapy is full of twists and turns, overlappings and reversals of both theory and method. And many of the terms I use—counterassumptive, counterprojective, performative—must be apologized for as "rebarbative," the adjective that the philosopher J. L. Austin so genially applied to his coinages. If I seem too strictly focused on verbal technique, I hope the reader and the practitioner will keep in mind that therapy, after all, is conducted in significant part through words.

Cambridge, Massachusetts   L. H.

Contents

Antecedents: Speaking to Absence   1

Empathic Language   9
  Finding the Other   11
  Imitative Statements   27
  Simple Empathic Statements   41
  Complex Empathic Statements   53
  Extensions   67

Interpersonal Language   81
  Good Management   83
  Projective Statements   97
  Counterassumptive Statements   111
  Counterprojective Statements   125

Performative Language   141
  Ideals and the Self   143
  Defending the Self   159

The Languages in Action   169

  Notes   185
  Acknowledgments   195
  Index   197

Making Contact

uses of language in psychotherapy

Antecedents: Speaking to Absence

Antecedents: Speaking to Absence

"Are you there?" A common enough question, and generally people don't ask it unless they expect the answer to be yes. But the answer therapists get, discounting hollow silence, is very often, "No, I'm not here." It is the most perplexing and disturbing situation in all of psychotherapy. My purpose in this book is to describe three forms of absence and the means to deal with them.

The first group of patients have hidden themselves away for protection from invasive others; many have in fact never developed an individuality of their own but have taken up an existence on the model of others. Empathic language provides the means to place the therapist *with* such patients (or the fragments of them to be found). A second form of absence involves patients who do not stay "there": they disappear into others and are often only detected by their effects on us. A frequent example is the "good patient," who can discover what pleases the therapist without even being told. Interpersonal language is the tool to establish a working distance from such invasive and obedient behavior. Finally, very many patients hardly exist at all. Their efforts at independent expression are met by criticism from both those around them and their own self-critical faculties—I call them the supine. Performative language aims at the liberation and development of the supine.

Broadly speaking we deal here with problems of isolation, domination, and submission, and the resulting distortions of character and situation. More closely speaking, this book is about speaking itself.

But why such emphasis on language and on these particular ways of talking? It might be useful to trace the beginnings of this work.

Thirty years ago one of my principal teachers, Ives Hendrick, laid down a challenge. He said that, when he had begun teaching psychiatry in the 1930s, the great task had been to keep doctors from talking too much in the therapeutic situation. This was so successfully accomplished by the 1950s that it was necessary to revive the use of speech and get them talking again. In historical terms, the method of free association had replaced the psychological examination. The influence of Freud persuaded many practitioners that access to deeper layers of mind occurred only through a steadfast attitude of listening and that healing action required the patient's transferring to the therapist feelings left over from childhood. At this point, clarification and interpretation of the transference phenomena usually followed, even though Freud himself was never too hopeful that such rational secondary process interventions could easily or decisively affect irrational emotional forces. Indeed, his psychology of the unconscious had undermined belief in the power of conscious, rational interventions.

So Hendrick was not able to teach us how we should speak, especially because most of the cases we were assigned little resembled the cases classified as "analyzable." Some teachers matched the difficulty of the cases with a comparably increased vigor of interpretation, almost like talking louder to someone hard of hearing. Yet it was difficult to imagine how this might lead to controllable results; interpretative success seemed to depend upon a high degree of cooperativeness or compliance on the part of the patient, which was either unreliably present or a sign of pathological submissiveness. My own experience as a psychoanalyst had convinced me that the most suitable cases for analysis were largely intact characterologically and their human situations amenable to change, so that the work could proceed in analytic anonymity and silence: these patients had within themselves the resources to deal with their conflicts once these conflicts had surfaced in the transference. Such cases, however, were not commonplace. Rather than exhibiting conflicts that could become self-adjusting, in the great majority of cases the relationship of psychic elements seemed more like examples of domination and submission, or of their isolation from one another. The imbalance of conflict or the separation of psychic elements implied that fresh approaches had to be introduced to right the imbalance or to bring the isolated elements together. The patients themselves did not appear to have such resources. How were these to be introduced?

Happily, I had two teachers gifted with an intuition that empowered them to speak effectively—Elvin Semrad, whom I knew at first hand, and Harry Stack Sullivan, whose writings I studied closely. Semrad had a remarkable gift for engaging absent people through empathic means very close to existential work, and Sullivan could break hostile stalemates arising interpersonally. I began to suspect that the answer to Hendrick's challenge lay at least partly in the hitherto unformulated languages that spring from the several schools of existential and interpersonal psychiatry. Would it be possible to address patients from the viewpoint of each of the schools?

The languages of the schools appear to be reflections of their basic perspectives. The languages are the instruments by which the perspectives are expressed. For example, the psychological examination and history taking of objective-descriptive psychiatry typically makes use of questions. The physician interrogates the patient, who must be able to understand the questions, ask them of himself, and report with accurate responses: a formidable array of internal reliabilities. In this school there is the sharpest subject-object differentiation—typically, *I* question *you*. The questions collect the symptoms and signs that define the sought-for disease state in the patient. For this reason, physicians sit opposite their patients with some object in between, a notepad to record accurately what is said or a desk to indicate professional objectivity.

In contrast, psychoanalysts utilize a language designed to elicit the freest possible associations, sitting behind the couch so that the desired reverie-like state will not be interrupted by the appearance and gestures of the analyst. Imperatives are the typical grammatical form: "Say whatever comes to mind" is the fundamental rule; even the repetitions, emphases, and urgings of less formal analytic requests suggest demands or entreaties. The whole work moves forward under a subtle command. At the same time, a subtle alliance is fostered. First-person plural statements, "We can see" or "We feel," ally analyst with patient for the observation of the patient.

Existential method depends heavily on rhetorical devices. These are expressive responses in keeping with the existential effort to be, or to empathize with, the patient. Empathic language carries out the purpose of entering the other's world, seeing that world through the other's eyes, and sharing the burdens and joys it contains. Here is the least subject-object separation. The characteristic sentence form involves the third-person impersonal singular: "It is awful" or "How awful it is."

What I have termed interpersonal and performative language characteristically employs declarative sentences. Statements of fact, hypothesis, or appraisal are offered for the patient's review. Third-person singular or plural forms, "He, She, They . . . ," direct attention away from the speaker and hearer to the social world. For the same reason, Sullivan sometimes sat beside his patients, more easily to look out at the interpersonal world where he located pathology. This position has an advantage that declarative statements also utilize: the interpersonal field can be cleared of the various projections each party brings to the transaction. (This is not to imply that every intervention by a therapist from any school is of only one order. Each of the schools encroaches readily on the other's turf, but there do seem to be prototypic forms for the respective intercessions.)

It also seemed to me that the different schools resolved themselves along refinements of basic psychological functions, and again the languages of the schools express these functions. The familiar names of the principal schools can even be replaced by those of the functions. Thus descriptive or medical psychological work makes primary use of perceiving. One of its great architects, Emil Kraepelin, was first and foremost a portraitist. From the thousands of patients he saw repeatedly over the course of his long clinical life, Kraepelin drew composite pictures that are recognizable to this day. Something similar could be said of Pierre Janet's work on the neuroses or Wilhelm Reich's description of character types. These are preeminent works of the *eye*.

In contrast, Freud's was a supremely explanatory gift. It is no accident that his materials were ideas, words, fantasies, always mental constructions, fed into and themselves constituting, by a kind of mental metabolism, the extraordinary body of his theories. Just as the Kraepelinian psychiatrist recognizes a disease entity and then attempts to affect it by medication or instruction, Freud performed an intellectual or cognitive task by interpreting and explaining to his subjects. The instrument here is the *head*.

Much interpersonal psychiatry seems the work of the *hand*. At least that function is suggested by other words—handle, manage, manipulate—so characteristic of, for example, Sullivan's interventions. In this work the observer participates because observation and contemplation alone miss the nimble, active sense of those clever hands. "Good management" is the term I use later, taken from D. W. Winnicott.

Empathic and much existential therapy is, above all, affective; the old-fashioned word to describe it is *heart*. The empathist feels. To the other schools, the existential enterprise seems lacking in sharpness, clear ideas, or practicality; in the existentialists' view, the disease doctors, analysts, and interpersonalists are without soul.

Perceiving, thinking, managing, feeling—such can be termed the specialties of the schools. Together they comprise a full response to the patient and point forward to the integrated psychotherapy I seek in this book. Of course the engine for this integration is not language alone; equally important is the therapist whose understanding becomes manifest in the language, an understanding both felt and abstract. The suggested language, experienced by the patient as understanding, makes contact with what are abstractly understood to be drives and internal structures. Words bring abstract understanding into relationship with experience; the persons involved become the conveyance. This process is similar to what engineering does with scientific principles. It translates them through the medium of the physical world.

Empathic Language

When a butterfly has to look like a leaf, not only are all the details of a leaf beautifully rendered, but markings mimicking grub-bored holes are generously thrown in. "Natural selection," in the Darwinian sense, could not explain the miraculous coincidence of imitative aspect and imitative behavior, nor could one appeal to the theory of "the struggle for life" when a protective device was carried to a point of mimetic subtlety, exuberance, and luxury far in excess of a predator's power of appreciation.

VLADIMIR NABOKOV

Finding the Other

All natural life abounds in versions of the chameleon. Even the most primitive creatures find ways to hide themselves for survival. The reason is simple: predation is the first and most terrifying fact of life. Humans have brought predation to profound levels of complexity and efficiency. These range from the attempted elimination of all creatures that threaten us, however great or small, to the harnessing of useful beasts in the laboratory or farm for our investigations and pleasures. This is not restricted to animals; human predation on our own species is equally widespread.

One result is that human disguises against predators are highly developed. There are minds so skittish and protective that we can compare them with small fish. They glide rapidly past us, quick to feel the movement of the water and changing color or shape at any hint of danger. A presence is almost impossible to secure— the elusive creature fears us. If we manage to catch and hold it, we may find it has altered its character to deceive.

A benign and gratifying example is the actor. His vivid or charming portrayal of a role allows the suspension of our disbelief. Biographies tell us that many great actors had miserable childhoods (Chaplin and Olivier come to mind). Their own identity or personality may be poorly developed, and they readily take on other personas. These are minds capable of the instant identifications called mimicry; they are able to refashion themselves after the example of others, seemingly without effort. Great actors live the part, as the expression goes. They imagine the gesture that accompanies the word and the word associated with the feeling. The whole sequence continues for an hour, an evening, years, or a lifetime. Some actors feel empty and lost without a part to play when they must return to their own apparently barren minds. It is also said that many psychopathic people who are imprisoned, unable to act on their impulses and move in the world, feel child-like and desolate.[1]

Human disguises against predation include that of the good patient. He or she is either amazingly docile or, even more difficult, so adept at discovering the therapist's expectations that what the therapist finds of the patient is only a mirror of his own wishes. Good patients often have no independent existence. They disappear into others and live there like parasites. It is a comfortable existence for many, one that is pleasing to the host, or hardly noticed until one or the other party grows restless and disappears. Other patients are only marginally present. Their central energies remain inside and they are able to reach only a little beyond themselves—hence Freud's term, the narcissistic neuroses. This failure is not restricted to people who are plainly psychotic. In fact, most psychotic people remain very attached to the world, although that attachment is dominated by fear. Many productive, apparently normal people do not have much interest in others, not even their spouses and children. The contacts they form with therapists are polite, intellectual, or manipulative, but without fire and blood. The whole psychoanalytic assumption of a treatment relationship that can mobilize the patient's deepest attachments and then change him by the examination of these attachments (what Freud called "the cure through love") collapses in the presence of such tepid, disinterested people.

It occurred to me that this phenomenon is even more widespread, that in a voluntary, intentional, and temporary form it constitutes a vital personal attribute. Every lecturer knows that behind the seemingly attentive and even enthusiastic faces of his audience are many absent minds. It is easy to recall one's own experience as listener, how the mind wanders to distant places, to people and matters more critical or interesting. In school we learn how to form these faces, nod occasionally, and check in often enough to be sure nothing new has been said. We can send our minds away, which may be the most important freedom we have.

Some patients do not have this freedom: they are afraid not to attend. Early in life parents had threatened any inattention with punishment, even claiming they knew what was on their child's mind and disapproving of it. As a result, the patients developed a permanent self-consciousness and self-watchfulness; they became imprisoned in paying attention. This may be one reason people "lose" their minds, as when the mind seems to speak to them from a corner of the room or from their stomachs, its contents scattered, leaving behind feelings of emptiness and desolation. Perhaps a mind that is under constant pressure and unable to send itself away for rest will escape of its own or explode.

Cannibalism and slavery are probably the oldest manifestations of human predation and submission. Although both are now discouraged, their continued existence in psychological forms demonstrates that civilization has achieved great success in moving from the concrete and physical to the abstract and psychological, while persisting in the same predatory purposes.

Take the matter of psychological slavery. Emil Kraepelin, the founder of modern descriptive psychiatry, utilized a test for what is called automatic obedience. This is today illustrated by the capacity of many schizophrenic people to hold a limb for long periods in whatever position the diagnostician places it. Kraepelin had a more precise, quantitative test. He took the physician's old standbys, tongue blade and straight pin, put the pin through the blade, and then told the patient to stick out his tongue. Most people will only hesitantly respond in such circumstances. Many schizophrenic people obey the command, receive the pin on their tongue, and only return tongue to mouth when told. Moreover, and still more incredibly, they will repeatedly accept the pin. This ←

[handwritten marginal note, right margin:] QUES: WOOULD THIS STILL BE FOUND TO BE CONSISTANT TODAY WITH THE INCREASE IN SELF ABUSE AND SELF ORUMUENTATION TREENDS (I.E: PIERCINGS EAR EYELID TONGUE CLIT ETC.)

is a quantitative test because the number of times the patient would continue to obey could be counted.

The biologists of schizophrenia may someday find the cerebral center for tongue extrusion and maybe even the lesion of it that prompts such bizarre behavior. In the meantime, we must suspect some element of psychological slavery in those called schizophrenic, with a parallel form of psychological mastery and tyranny in those close to them. Automatically obedient patients sometimes do the opposite of what is asked, but they are still enslaved. Whether it is possible for human beings to continue existing under such conditions is uncertain. Perhaps some can. We are only now beginning to learn what happens to people who are controlled by the different forms of slavery.[2]

Can the living, talking, interacting patient avoid bringing something of himself to the therapist? Even his disguises are his own. Yet how do we know? In drug clinics, addicts often submit someone else's urine for testing because their own would expose the continuing habit. Comparable substitutions are a psychological commonplace. Often the psychotherapeutic patient does not realize he is substituting another's substance. The most dramatic example is the phenomenon of *folie à deux*.[3] Generally this occurs in a passive person who falls under the influence of a characteristically active, older paranoid personality and is transformed into the dominant person's image. It can be done so subtly that the passive individual feels he is the other and will spout strange delusions as his own.

In old Chinese medicine, the patient would stand behind a screen and hold up a doll, pointing to where the pain was, thus preserving modesty. I encountered one patient who resembled a mannequin; she was her own doll. Sadly, this was a more profound hiding than in the Chinese anecdote. My patient could hardly point to where the pain was, and I had to go in search of it.

The most famous example of deceptive psychiatric patients involved one of the cleverest doctors who ever lived. Jean-Martin Charcot was more than an important contributor to internal medicine and the discoverer of several neurological conditions; he also was one of the principal forerunners of psychoanalysis. His account of the symptoms and signs of hysteria, however, is a model of this kind of deception. Hysterical and epileptic patients lived together in the Saltpêtrière asylum, where Charcot was the great luminary. The young hysterics would hold the epileptics when they fell and nurse them during their postseizure confusions. Here is Charcot's description of hysterical attacks:

> The patient loses consciousness and the paroxysm proper begins. It is divided into four periods which are quite clear and distinct. In the first, the patient executes certain epileptiform convulsive movements. Then comes the period of great gesticulations of salutation, which are of extreme violence, interrupted from time to time by an arching of the body which is absolutely characteristic, the trunk being bent bow fashion, sometimes in front (emprosthotonos), sometimes backward (opisthotonos), the feet and head alone touching the bed, the body constituting the arch, during which he utters words and cries in relation with the sad delerium and terrifying visions which pursue him.[4]

Janet wrote that suggestibility was the most reliable sign of hysteria, and what Charcot saw was, in part, a mimicking of epilepsy.[5] There also is evidence that students of Mesmer, the magnetizers, were loose on the Saltpêtrière wards, producing the convulsive emotional crises that they thought curative.[6] Charcot wanted to describe a discrete, well-demarcated disease, as he had done so brilliantly in the neurological realm: hysteria, sometimes called the great imitator, obliged. Let the designers of diagnostic systems beware.

The point is, when an individual has been reduced to obedience and disobedience, assumes often impenetrable disguises, keeps his mind from us, or has altogether lost it, his real self may be difficult to find.

Therapeutic Empathy

In the Japanese movie *Kagemusha,* a warlord is about to die; in order to secure a period of peace before the succession, a double is put in his place. The imposter so closely resembles the warlord that he deceives everyone except the warlord's concubines. They have intimately "known" the warlord in the act of love, and they do not find the same person in the imposter.

One clinical equivalent of this knowing intimacy is empathy. My thesis here is that the most certain way of knowing when a person is present, of finding the other, lies in the ability to empathize with that person.

A young man came to me complaining of intense burning feelings over much of his skin. He claimed that, some weeks before, an unnamed man had implanted radioactive material in his brain, which caused the burning. In his childhood and youth, the patient had been poorly served by his father. Perhaps as a result, he had repeatedly formed devoted attachments to unreliable older men, the latest of whom had rejected him shortly before the skin irritation began. In addition, both his mother and stepmother had forbidden him to return to their homes. All of this he recounted calmly.

I tried to attune myself closely to what he may have felt and translated these emotions into words: "That must have hurt!" These remarks were spoken with force. When he referred to the rejection by his mothers, I even experienced a burning ragelike feeling on my own skin. In turn, he spoke more forcefully of the occurrences, and I again felt the burning, although much attenuated. The patient then remarked that the burning sensation was gone. I'm not saying that my reaction is typical or generally possible—only that empathy is a capacity to participate in or experience another's sensations, feelings, thoughts, or movements.[7] Finding the other, therefore, means finding appropriate sensations, feelings, thoughts, and movements: these are the data of empathic work.

The therapist can distinguish between active and passive empathy. In active empathy one searches out the other. There is a "bold swinging . . . into the life of the other," to use Martin Buber's colorful phrase,[8] a verbal expression of what one intuits the other is feeling. In this way, sometimes even catatonic people can be reached.

The balancing catatonic, for instance, was completely rigid, mute and unresponsive until someone joined her in her balancing act as if dancing. All of a sudden, she was transformed; one could hardly recognize her as the same patient. She told us everything we wanted to know about her love affair and her life-story, with complete clarity, like any healthy person. We were able to repeat the experiment several times before the increasing severity of her catatonia made it impossible.[9]

Waiting for such a transformation is usually in vain, but by putting what one imagines into gestures, words, or feelings, it is possible to touch and stir the patient, even to the point of some gradual liberation.

Conversely, passive empathy is a waiting, sentient attitude, echoing some of the patient's statements and, above all, supporting and reflecting his emotions. Carl Rogers has called it a nondirective or client-centered therapy. The earliest observations of affective empathy were not made so purposefully, of course; changes in the observer's responsiveness sprang up spontaneously, and empathy was inadvertent. Best known was *praecoxgefuhl,* the eerie feeling one gets in the presence of the schizophrenic person,[10] sometimes accompanied by erection of the small hairs at the back of the observer's neck. Your blood runs cold. Horror movies and the great tales of terror, like James's *The Turn of the Screw,* can produce the same sensation. You want to run but feel caught, as in many nightmares.

There are also "group signs." When entering a conference room after a depressed patient has been interviewed, you can usually read the diagnosis off the forlorn faces of the interviewers. In contrast, the psychopathic subject leaves them divided—the presenting therapist has been "taken in" and defends his patient against the derision of the group. Hysterical female patients cause a different split: men defend them, and women scoff. (All of this can be called "fossil diagnosis" because the patient leaves a characteristic imprint behind.)

Contagion of every affect has been reported by therapists: anxiety, depression, anger, excitement, ecstasy, even affectlessness.[11] One often feels empty and drifting after contact with chronically psychotic people; nothing from the interview can be recalled. You move cautiously, lethargically, as if a spell had been cast. The transmission of hysterical excitement and behavior is an old observation in the psychology of crowds. It sets in motion a charismatic invasiveness, as the leader shares the dramatic and hyperbolic feelings so characteristic of hysteria. Social gatherings flourish in the artificial glitter of manic and hysterical people. As a result, no wise hostess invites guests who are even a little depressed.[12]

Often if the therapist of a depressed person feels depressed himself, the patient improves. It is as if the therapist has relieved the patient of his despondency. It is a dangerous sign if a worker does not become depressed while caring for a suicidal patient; he may not have come close enough to aid the suffering person.

Sullivan once claimed that he could recognize a homosexual by a tightening of the anal sphincter. A foolish listener asked, "Whose?" as if anyone but a proctologist knew much about the patient's sphincter. There is also Hendrick's assertion that a male therapist will feel scrotal and penile movement in the presence of a hysterical woman.

These phenomena are evidence of the active, invasive functioning of the patient's mind. Manic patients produce excited wards, and paranoiacs will argue with argumentative therapists. The recorder of a depressed person's history does not wonder why it is one of regrets, mistakes, broken relationships and hopes. We feel we are in the presence of a real other, however incompletely or temporarily manifest. As a result, clinical work moves through an underworld of strong emotional tones that unobtrusively shape and move us. The therapist has to grasp these forces and turn them to clinical advantage.

Tests of Empathy

One reads the extent of empathic contact off the dial of one's reactions. Motor empathy has already been described in the case of the balancing catatonic. I found another, literal illustration of this in a photograph depicting a group of people who twist in unison while observing a pole-vaulter clear the bar. The empathic clinician sometimes finds himself crossing his legs or gesturing in unison with a patient.

Affective empathy is the experience of the patient's feeling state by the therapist. It is a test easily enough made. We determine the other's feeling state by observing his expressions, tone of voice, posture, and the thousand objective expressions of affect the body produces, including autonomic ones. We also note the content of speech. Sad people depreciate themselves, regret the past, and despair of the future; happy people express the opposite. Angry people vent their rage: the prototypic statement is "God damn the world!" In contrast, flat people lack definable content; their speech wanders, is fragmented, hard to remember. Having made these determinations of affect, we then compare the result with our feelings. In this second step we have the advantage of feeling our own emotions directly, yet in both cases we can note the content of speech.

The tests of successful cognitive and perceptual empathy have a startling clarity. Cognitive empathy is best measured by the therapist's attempting inwardly to complete the patient's sentences. The more closely the therapist can match what the patient then says, the closer he is to the patient. Old people who have lived many years together speak in half sentences, in part because their empathic awareness is so great. People in love often do too. Again: you take the empathic reading off the dial of your own reactions.

Perceptual empathy means seeing something for the first time. Matisse is rumored to have told his students, "Go out and see a flower for the first time." The point is to see without presuppositions or expectations, the habitual baggage of perception. To see in this way is to see according to the fundamental rule of existential work, the psychological-phenomenological reduction: "In the presence of a phenomenon (whether it be an external object or a state of mind), the phenomenologist uses an absolutely unbiased approach; he observes phenomena as they manifest themselves and only as they manifest themselves."[13] In Rollo May's words, what is sought is "a sudden, sometimes powerful experience of here is a new person, an experience that normally carries with it an element of surprise."[14]

Our changing perceptions signal one of the difficulties of evaluating patients' progress in psychotherapy. Often we do not know whether changes in their appearance are real or a function of progressively seeing the patients in a fresh way. Sometimes the two seem related: previously locked into the world's (or his own) perception of him, the patient can change when seen in a new way. In my experience, a bit-by-bit reperception of a gradually emerging person is more common than a sudden, new seeing of the whole person. Again, the reality and the perception seem often interlocked, so that we are puzzled as to which changes first. Nevertheless, many patients are not perceivable in a fresh way. No doubt this is the failure of the observer to be sufficiently perceptive. Others shine forth immediately as they are. Some patients, however, may not be freshly perceivable because there is no distinct, unique person to be perceived. With imposters, what is commonly seen are the lineaments of a role they have assumed, and there may be nothing else to see. As a result, empathy will be very difficult or impossible.

To those for whom the word "test" denotes chemical or arithmetic testing, a sharply defined procedure with a numerical result, these psychological tests must be disappointing. The historically minded reader will be able to recall when medicine was dependent on such testing procedures as percussion and auscultation, when the physician determined the boundaries of fluid accumulation or the size of the heart by tapping his finger on the patient's chest wall. Such methods were a central part of the physician's skills until quite recently and offer a nice analogy to where psychiatry now stands. Just as the physician tapped his finger or put his ear as close as possible to the heart, the psychiatrist uses himself as an instrument of testing, his own affects, his own sense of closeness, his own movements to and from the patient.

Time and Space

To find another, you must enter that person's world. The empathic visitor then discovers what he has taken for granted in his own world: that it is a world of particular time and space.

We divide what Minkowski terms "lived time" into the past, present, and future.[15] Empathic reports suggest a psychopathology of time, meaning that the experiences of past, present, and future can be deranged.[16] Of course any such alleged derangement supposes a normal experience of time. The normal person, or more appropriately, the ideal or authentic person, experiences himself as growing toward the future.[17] This is not to say the future is a fixed point to be reached, that one ever "makes it"; rather, the future is the site of both anticipation and the unexpected, planning and the changing of plans. This predominant orientation toward a changing future also means a fluid or unfixed past, because the past is continually being reassessed as one moves into the future. The present, standing between the past and future, is the occasion of building; in the present the past is developed into the future. Thus the present signals that one can never successfully break past from future; the past nourishes the future.

It is possible for one to lose present, past, or future. In depression the future is lost, and the past becomes fixed, immovable, bad, the place of irredeemable mistakes. In contrast, the past can be lost as one soars maniacally into an unreal future. Lists are made in order to occupy and control the future before it happens. Anticipating becomes a disease when it merges present with future: there is nothing in the present except this futuring. In the first case, the actual present is lost to the past; in the second it has vanished into the future. In either instance, there is no building.

Both past and future can be lost to the present as well. One lives for the moment, afraid to look back or ahead. One surrenders to a mindless busyness which is not building, or to sensation—for example, gluttony or resistance to gluttony. One can also yield to the contemplation of motionlessness, which has much in common with many schizophrenic states of changelessness, hope-lessness, and flatness.[18]

People exist not only in time but also in their bodies, which in turn exist in the world. The category of space, therefore, in-cludes bodyhood and the world. The body is in the world and on the world; we can feel rooted. This is sometimes a heavy feeling, as when the past seems heavy in depression, or the body when it is fat or inert. Or the rootedness may be lively, with a sense of living connections, just as the past can relate productively to the future. The metaphor is revealing: as living roots grow, search out water and food, and thus create change, so human roots nourish and cause change.

Disorders of space are among the commonest that human beings experience. Perhaps the most prevalent of these is the fear of heights, where one feels unrooted, able or even eager to fall. Existential workers suggest that the more deeply rooted one is, the greater the loss of grounding space needed to precipitate the fear. Yet everyone should be afraid to fall; the security of ground-ing space is only transient, as anyone who lives in earthquake country knows. One result is that the psychopathology of space includes both those who fear too readily and those who do not fear enough.

It is often said that the fear of open spaces originates in a fear of what those open spaces can bring. Over the rim of the earth may be marching enemies or typhoons—above all, the unex-pected. This is the nature of both space and future time, and much of the past as well: to contain the unexpected. I suggest that unexpectedness is the existential equivalent of the Freudian unconscious, or what physical science calls the unknown. The expected can be discounted, as they say in the commercial markets, while against the unexpected there is usually confusion, denial, and turmoil, the sense of being thrown. It is the slow translation of the unexpected into the expected that constitutes much of wisdom. Even death comes to be expected, thereby losing its terror.

The sense of being thrown is fundamental to human experience because the random, and its capacity to throw us, occurs at the very start of life and never altogether ends. Such emphasis on the random appears to pit existential thought against science. In fact, this stress on the random is merely a reminder of how infrequently science has been able to predict and control human experience. Human life remains largely "thrown": the sperm into the uterus, the child into the family, the adult into marriage and society. For all we know and choose, each of these fundamental steps contains elements unpredictable and therefore, from the viewpoint of experience, random.

Perhaps it is for this reason that many small children delight in being thrown into the air, if they are firmly caught again: is a fundamental fear being met and mastered? There is a cruel story about a father who deliberately drops his child on the last throw, saying, "Now you know not to trust anyone." He is saying that there is no value in basic trust. The father is partly correct— psychiatrists probably practice more off the too-trusting than from the too-suspicious. Still, it is a cruel joke because we suspect the child may become so fearful of being thrown that she cannot allow herself to be thrown into the world at all.

Space is not only a source of unexpectedness, but also where we experience size. The physically large and small can be looming and overwhelming or creeping and invasive. Bodily size can immediately generate feelings of importance or grossness. Yet it is in an unexpected quarter that spatiality reveals perhaps its strongest hold on human experiencing. There is a line from E. E. Cummings, "As small as a world and as large as alone."[19] Being part of a human world is experienced as a closeness, an intimacy, a bounding of the world, while to be alone is often to feel the limitlessness of the world. The verse is only superficially a paradox, since whatever relates to and reaches us necessarily defines a world that is otherwise immense. Even the extraordinary distances covered in space travel bring the universe closer: a large part of what closeness means is this capacity to reach or touch. Reaching and rootedness are therefore only different words for the same experience of connectedness. One emphasizes exploring, touching; the other, settlement and integration.

The spatial world of the other is defined by the extent and

quality of its connectedness. While the present connects past and future, defining the extent and quality of a person's connections between past and future, human presence connects the body and the world. Spatial connections stream across that boundary of presence between the body and the world. Thus, when we admire someone's presence, we are connecting ourselves to that person; when we cherish that presence, we feel a desire for the person that links us intimately.

Similarly, when we know that time seems to stop in depression, we can more easily put ourselves in the world of the depressed other. It is a dramatic experience to share the flat timelessness of many chronically schizophrenic people, and then to watch them light up in recognition of your sudden presence in their lives. The patients feel found, and not in the sense of found out or criticized. Moreover, the recognition of time's suspension may suggest a time when it is not suspended, when life can start to move.

The operative phrase for this finding the other is Buber's "imagining the real." The conditions of empathy are the therapist's power to imagine the experience of the other and then to express it. The phrase is striking because it conflates two ideas usually opposed, the imaginary and the real; it is the unreal we think we must imagine. It is only in the grasping of an unknown reality that imagination is called for unequivocally. When the boot hits the rock, even when another personality is encountered, if that personality presents itself fully and forcefully, then imagination is at most called for to amplify or complete what we encounter. In the penetration of the unknown, however, this psychological order is largely reversed. Einstein remarked that no amount of empirical fact could have led to the complicated equations of his theories.[20] The central requirement was the imaginative or hypothetical. Similarly, when a personality cannot present itself or does so incompletely or falsely, our only recourse is to the imagination, made still more compelling by the realization that even the most vivid personality (and sometimes, one suspects, especially the most vivid personality) may be presenting a false front that needs to be tested for its authenticity.

In *Kagemusha* the imposter played the part assigned him. The powers behind the throne manipulated him; certainly the role he played would have meant nothing if the powers had not needed him, and if most of the others had not reinforced him. What might we call the concubines? Were they psychoanalysts who could discover his sexual wishes to be different from the warlord's? Or were they existentialists who sensed in the superb actor the absence of a person to be with? Each would imagine something different to be real: the needs of the kingdom, the sexual wishes, the person.

The imposter's wishes could have been very real: to save his life, to be king, to have the concubines, perhaps even someday to be his own person. We would do different therapies if the imposter resented giving up his spurious kingship, or if he could not satisfy the concubines, or if he were tired of pretending to be king. The first order of clinical business is to find the other, however distant, absent, or confused, who may one day tell us what he does want. This is what gives empathy its frequent priority, allowing us to become the patient's other, supporting his or her search for what is wanting, and providing guidance in how we find it. The language of psychotherapeutic empathy expresses states of mind, the most rudimentary through imitative statements, and multiple and conflicting states of mind through simple and complex empathic statements. Any thoroughgoing search for the other also implies an exploration of the other's world.

Yet truth, like love and sleep, resents
Approaches that are too intense.

W. H. AUDEN

Imitative Statements

Cognitive empathy, where the therapist silently completes the patient's sentences, is both the most precise and the least used method of testing. It is a form of mind reading. The therapist who shares a patient's world listens, at the same time, to the patient and to his own resonances with the patient. He can test immediately and exactly the extent of that resonance by the closeness of his own inner voice to the spoken words of the patient. It is most accurate when the patient uses familiar and habitual phrasings—others are elusive. Yet, in fact, reading minds with a measure of accuracy is generally possible.

What I term imitative statements are nothing more than these inner voices of the therapist speaking out loud for the patient, what is called "doubling" in psychodrama and work with children. Thus: "How can I decide?" might be said to the doubtful person; "What hope is there?" to the depressed one; or "Where does one find the courage?" to fearful ones. There are as many imitative statements as there are thoughts to be shared, but for clinical use they sort into types that have specific purposes.

The first objective is to indicate that the therapist is with the patient, specifically with those who both need someone and yet find it difficult to have anyone close. To such individuals, imi-

27

tative statements must above all be *bland*. The goal is to comfort by our presence, not to startle by our prescience. Not everyone knows that minds can be read or that only a few people are so creative and unique that their thoughts could surprise anyone. Many people are deeply private; they believe their thoughts should never be known, often not so much out of shame or fear but rather out of a sense of possession. These are people whose self-possession has been eroded from the start; they have been forced to move further and further into themselves, like a defeated populace retreating to mountain or jungle country. When we read minds, we are once again threatening self-possession.

The idea that we may or may not possess ourselves is at one moment obvious and at the next obscure. It is obvious because self-possession is easily recognizable, as in the form of poise, or in the lack of it when we become frazzled or out of control. Its obscurity stems from the fact that the self is as much a possessor as a possession, and because the notion of self is itself so elusive.[1]

It was once common to speak of being possessed, as by the devil. The goal of treatment or exorcism was to return the self to the self or, in some formulations, to God. Today we refer to people as self-centered, or full-of themselves, and this is another object of treatment. We see in this contrast the difficulty of such concepts as self-possession or self-centeredness: we want the self to possess itself but not to center on itself; the self is to be both inside and outside itself, and yet to *be* itself. All these conflicting claims come out in therapy, when we must seek to approach the self without invading it.

The uncertainty of self-possession begins early because parents think they "own" their children. Everyone speaks of "their" children just as they refer to their houses and cars. In fact, children can be disowned, both legally and less formally, as when a disappointed father tells "his" wife to correct "her" child. I can recall the christening of one of "my" children, during which the baby dropped her rattle. The minister retrieved the toy and handed it back, saying, "This belongs to you, Emily, but you do not belong to your parents, but to God." It was a salutary remark, but the lesson is more often painfully learned, for instance when divorced couples have to share children with stepparents or when adoptive parents must share them with birth parents. Shortly I will describe a young woman whose mother, angry at an aloof daughter, said, "Your sister is so ungrateful. Thank God I've got you." Most children do not like being possessed and withdraw from people whom they perceive as invasive or possessive. This suggests that the sense of self develops early. But some children do not seem free to indicate their displeasure and so are all the more easily possessed.

Empathic statements, if insufficiently tested for the accuracy of empathy, can easily be used to force patients to feel what the therapist believes they feel or should feel. Many patients, like the poorly protected children, do not indicate their displeasure or may not even feel it. In such a case, a more neutral empathy is called for. This first class of imitative statements does not challenge, impress, or reach into what is private and defended. Instead it increases or secures the other's self-possession. The statements are like white flags that contesting armies fly to signal the other's safety. One of the themes of this book is "giving someone freedom." These first imitative statements are beginning efforts in the cause. Their purpose is to offer oneself to someone for *their* purpose.

Approaching Softly

Jeanne, a nineteen-year-old woman, entered treatment because of anxiety and purposelessness.[2] She rarely attended her college classes, smoked a great deal of pot, and did whatever her crowd did. She was an attractive, well-off girl who took no joy in showing off her considerable good looks. When she was not being compliant, she seemed absent-minded and distant.

Jeanne described her father as a wealthy lawyer and her mother as depressed. For as far back as she could remember, each of them had complained to her about the other. In the last few years this had grown progressively more irritating and embarrassing. She said her father gave her everything she wanted and frequently asked if she were happy, but he hardly existed for her except as a source of money. Her mother disapproved of his lavishness but was generous with praise herself. She wanted to know everything her daughter did and thought, frequently bought duplicate dresses so they could look alike, and was overjoyed if Jeanne dated the "right" boys. There was an older sister, who was abrupt, overbearing, and had little to do with the family; Jeanne felt deserted by her.

Jeanne recalled that since before adolescence she had wanted to be pretty and to meet the right man. Her mother repeatedly assured her that this would happen, but so far it had not and she was puzzled and annoyed by her boyfriends. She described them as either lunging at her or keeping their distance. She did not seem to realize that she had in fact become quite beautiful and that boys were both drawn to and repelled by her mixture of beauty, absent-minded hauteur, and compliance. Without knowing it, she had become the fairy princess she and her mother had wanted her to be.

Jeanne had a definite "identity" as a beautiful rich girl who could have anything she wanted and needed only to await her Prince Charming. Nevertheless, she was not in possession of herself, that is, hers were incomplete and unacknowledged goals and unaccepted facts. She did not feel beautiful and could only secretly dream of being both beautiful and well loved. Early in treatment she exposed this "rich and beautiful" identity to me, but she was also hiding herself away. It was like being with a mannequin.

A simple, direct approach would have been, "What's the matter with being rich and beautiful? Come out and enjoy it." We then might have analyzed any conflicts she had about those qualities and other goals. In fact, the conflict was not between the patient's wishes and any prohibiting agencies. It turned out that Jeanne was glad to be rich and beautiful; her parents' wanting her to be so did not stop her from enjoying the condition. The difficulty seemed to lie elsewhere. She did not experience herself at all; she was also a mannequin to herself. This woman was like many favored people who have become their money or their beauty and have no capacity left to enjoy them.

Why didn't she experience herself? Possibly this was also a

function of conflict between parts of her mind. Yet there was little or no evidence of conflict, unless the inexperience of self is evidence itself. There was no apparent guilt within herself or the family. They felt, probably correctly, that wealth and beauty were what most people wanted. Even the usually charged theme of being more beautiful than the mother was discussed, at times even laughed about, by both of them. It certainly could not be that she was without any oedipal disturbances, but there was little evidence of them, definitely none in the sexual area, where she enjoyed herself. Sexuality was where she felt most alive.

One day Jeanne seemed especially still and distant. I mused aloud, "What *is* one supposed to do?" To my surprise, she crisply replied, "Right!" and after a long pause, "I don't know what to do. I *never* know what to do." I had put myself in the midst of her uncertainty, verbalized it for her, and shared her desperation by my tone. At the same time, there was no implication that she should know or decide, as many ways of calling attention to her indecision might have suggested. She then described talking to a dean about her courses. She had pretended that she knew and liked the courses, that they meant something to her. In fact, she seldom attended any classes.

"The only things *I* know I want are being beautiful and married," I said. Now I was approaching less softly. Again she responded very crisply, "Right!" and seemed to relax. I added, "What else was I supposed to be?" "Nothing," she said. "Father, of course, was different," I said. With a rising sarcastic inflection and a big smile, she said, "Was he ever!" I didn't want her to feel too sorry for herself in this typical woman's position, so I added, "A woman's lot." There was another pause until she said, in a crescendo of surprise and revelation to us both, "My mother never does anything!"

When I first met Jeanne, she was infatuated with a boy whose behavior puzzled and depressed her. He would approach her, say something friendly, then rush away. Once or twice he stayed long enough to sit down with her, and she became dizzy with excitement. Afterwards, when he disappeared for two weeks, she was despondent. Jeanne did not know that some people behave strangely around the rich and beautiful, often approaching and rapidly retreating, as this boy did. It is as if they are afraid to stay too close to the flame.[3]

Naturally Jeanne had been unsettled by the boy's comings and goings and was now upset by what she regarded as a rejection. I guessed that, for her, this was the prince that mother had promised, rather than the vain young man I suspected. However, this was only conjecture because she would not describe anything about him except his movements. He had a way of psychologically disappearing that was as complete as her own. Simple empathic statements, such as "It is awful to be left," did not accomplish much; she would get teary-eyed, then fall silent. She was supposed to be happy, she thought, and sadness was not acceptable.

My question "Can he love me?" caught her interest. My next "Can I love him?" was startling at first, followed by "Why is he so elusive?" "*Aren't* I beautiful?" seemed to baffle and then delight her. These were not my questions to her, but as if posed by her; they were important because she was confused and questioning. I closed with, "I just hope he's worth your while," which placed me squarely on Jeanne's side and raised questions about the boy. Then she told me she had loved him, would have done anything for him. But she had not experienced his interest in her and could not see or feel herself in the interaction. Again, to herself, she hardly existed. The depression lifted as she remembered more about the boy. She drew back and became less subservient. Later, when Jeanne had more confidence, she gave him some of his own approach/avoidance medicine, which let her see at close hand how fearful he was, and how adoring. It was a sweet revisit. Still later, she became almost worldly-wise. I sensed a great coming out. I had to laugh when she told me she had uncovered a "psychopath" who was only interested in her looks and her father's money. She left him for good, after a long, expensive dinner, before the bill arrived; he had expected her to pay.

Early on, Jeanne's intelligence was obvious, along with something still very faint that was generous and down-to-earth. It seemed to peek out from behind the mannequin. Later I will describe the means used to foster those qualities. Here it is important to emphasize how vulnerable she was while emerging. Perhaps Jeanne's parents had sensed this, hence their oppressive protection of her. This could partly explain the father's often puzzling behavior; he told her she was very bright but would not allow her to do anything for herself. It does not explain the full extent of his control, though, because he had a similar attitude toward the mother and behaved toward the whole family much as he did in his many successful financial dealings, with a commanding power over details. In a business society like ours, it may be inevitable that paternal and financial authority should coalesce to the detriment of many family members. Jeanne was only an extension of the father's business holdings, and a younger version of the mother and her hopes. What little she was doing at the start of our work was only a function of her father's or mother's purposes. This state of protected ownership made her supremely naive. In turn, this naiveté made her susceptible to her parents' ownership and encouraged further protectiveness.

Here she was—beautiful, rich, intelligent, amiable—yet she spent most of her time alone. One reason became clear when she mentioned a boy who had told her she was beautiful. Jeanne's roommate advised her not to believe him. In fact Jeanne had accepted the observation as a plain statement of fact. This was a part of herself she had come to recognize and acknowledge, and openly acknowledge it she did, on several occasions. As a result, one of two things would happen. Some boys thought she was vain and disliked her for it. Others were taken aback by her openness, felt challenged, and retreated in fear. She seldom had more than two or three dates with any boy.

Her roommate was correct: Jeanne was not supposed to believe the boy. The conventional response would be to act as if the praise were mere flattery, part of a courting ritual, which gives both parties time to address their fears and ambivalences. In contrast, the patient went straight to the point. As she emerged from behind her mask, she did so openly and without protection. She emerged naked.[4]

Helping the Naked

In 1920 Milena Jesenska-Pollak wrote about Franz Kafka, "Frank does not have the capacity for living . . . He is absolutely incapable of lying, just as he is incapable of getting drunk. He possesses not the slightest refuge. For that reason he is exposed to all those things against which we are protected. He is like a naked man among a multitude who are dressed."[5] I once met a famous man who provides a useful contrast to Kafka and the patients I am describing. This man tries to be real and does everything he imagines real people do, being sincere, friendly, brave, simple, even a little foolish at times. Yet he does not seem at all real to me. It is not because he is so inhumanly good and does nothing wrong. Rather, it is that the whole effort is undertaken with an eye on himself: it is an act.

The contrast is useful because it underscores the desirability of being neither naked nor overdressed. Psychiatrists treasure patients who reveal themselves, and often these therapists reinforce dangerous innocence by their pleased responses to the revelations. They also overvalue patients who respect their interpretations, overlooking the depressive self-depreciation that may make the patient welcome bad news. The point is that patients need to strike a balance between being connected and self-protective.

One thirty-five-year-old man I treated was as naked at the start of psychotherapy as Jeanne had become during its course. Francis had learned honesty, obedience, duty, and directness from his mother and grandmother, and he had been a victim of these qualities ever since. This man encountered the worst difficulties when he fell in love; he called himself "lost." By this Francis meant that he felt himself disappear into his beloved, merge with her, become dependent on her every mood or gesture, and then resentful of his helplessness. He explained that this was just what he had felt with his mother and was the reason he had left home at sixteen. "She would never let me do anything; I'd start and she would finish. She wanted me to be very good, understand and help everyone." There was no disagreeing with her either; she would simply leave the room. He either felt dependent and directed or alone and abandoned. She had not let him separate, and he could not find his own purposes and personality. He remained the unconscious instrument of her saintly goals.

Many people become patients when they fall in love. A good part of the remaining therapeutic practice is with those who cannot fall in love. Falling in love is dangerous because it is like a psychosis and therefore can easily become one. The lover misperceives his beloved, pours himself into the beloved, goes about in a daze, and is often jealous to the point of paranoia. Poets call love blind or foolish or mad. An old adage cautions to keep your eyes open before marriage and half shut afterwards. This is wise advice, prompting that sad line of Pope's, "They dream in courtship but in wedlock wake."

Many people become patients when they fall in love because they literally fall; they cannot dive or control the fall.[6] My patient fell back into the arms of his mother, back into dependence. For a while Francis' girlfriends would be flattered and attentive, until his demands increased. Then they became frightened and withdrew, quite shattering Francis. He had literally given himself away, both his possessions and his mind. This was long before I met him. He had avoided love affairs after that and turned to therapy, but the same thing happened there. He undertook the work enthusiastically. The therapist was pleased and eager. The patient increased his demands, telephoned too often, and refused to leave the sessions; the therapist withdrew. Francis was hospitalized.

He then spent three years with a therapist who was reportedly cold and distant. "He never did anything for me." Yet in that unpromising setting, Francis grew stronger. Although he did not venture back into love, he had several rewarding relationships, and his career progressed. This patient came to me complaining about the distant therapist and his own feelings of loneliness. He soon showed the two sides of himself. When I empathized, or was even slightly sympathetic, he cried, seeming to dissolve into gentle self-pity. He could have climbed into my lap. Then, when I was cool, he complained, "You're making me worse. I don't know why I see you." He became the unassisted isolate who must set things right on his own.

Francis was not a difficult man to find—the problem here was to establish a working distance. His presence was distinct, almost enveloping. I was confused only because he showed such contrasting sides: the close, helpless dependence and the distant, disappointed rage. It was as if his mind consisted of a substance extraordinarily sensitive to both hot and cold, having the lowest possible boiling point and the highest possible freezing point. Only a small gradient in between was available to me. Of course his difficulty was the same. On an everyday basis he felt either pulled into very friendly people or completely frozen out by others. Often he could hardly hear what people said, especially if they praised or criticized him, because he was moving so rapidly toward or away from them.

Everything seemed to depend on moderating my distance from him. I wanted to be close enough so that we could form a bond sufficient to make separation meaningful, but not so close that separation would be impossible. I would have to remain physically and psychologically present when he complained, but my closeness should not be choking. The safest intervention in this situation was the use of imitative statements.

It was essential that Francis continue to experience my presence, even when attacking me; otherwise it would have been easy for him to imagine that he had destroyed me or disgraced himself. His perceptions were keen, so I frequently had to acknowledge my own ineffectiveness. This was performed confidently, to demonstrate I had survived. I learned to expect an hourly ten to fifteen minutes of such lambasting, and set myself to endure it, sometimes even to the point of enjoyment. (It was all good practice for family life.)

It was just as important to gauge my closeness. The yearning little boy could only be allowed out for limited periods and then had to be gently cuffed. He said he could cry forever, and I believed him. If I said "Why can't I be loved?" the little boy would come out, sobbing. "What can one expect of this bloody world?" said tartly, a little coolly, would send him footdragging back. "What can one expect of this bloody world?" had another purpose as well. Friendliness always snared him, and Francis became an instant slave. He had to learn whether the friendliness was real or manipulative, to raise that boiling point. This might be accomplished by fulfilling part of his need for closeness, but I also wanted to hold him back. It was necessary for him to judge people more carefully and not be taken in. This was a man who had been wounded often and had felt the world's pitilessness many times, but he was the least cynical of humans. Hopefulness existed right next to his angry despair.

Such a condition is often found in patients whose parents have either held them very close or been very distant. The childish, grandiose expectations these people have of their parents do not wear away, but the wearing away is necessary because through it comes the discovery that parents are ordinary people. Diminishing overblown expectations requires give and take in the middle distance. My patient had never experienced this with his parents. Francis didn't have to learn to trust; he had to learn not to trust. He had to surrender his expectations of a perfectly safe closeness. He would cry thinking of it, sad at relinquishing the dream of paradise. Sometimes he would subtly build others up, in the hope that their strength could give him safety. So discreet was the building that the others would not credit him. Often they would use their new strength to put him down. His innocence and trustfulness simply brought out the predatory in others. A Russian proverb says, "Be a lamb and the wolf will appear." I had to resist too, as Francis tendered himself to me for penetrating interpretations.

Late in our work, he startled me by saying that two friends had learned in law school what he was trying to learn now. He said they had been taught to simulate, to take any side and argue instantly and aggressively the case put to them. It was exactly what he could not do. He was either up front and naked or hidden away. The result was that not only did I feel helpless to interpret, but I could barely ask for information; this opened him up further and encouraged him to give still more of himself away. It would be better then to acknowledge my stupidity and not saddle him with the burden of once again making someone else look good. By not interpreting, by not asking for information, by remarking on my stupidity, I could give him enough distance for his safety and enough of my presence to continue contact. The goal was a middle distance: Francis was to have the hitherto unknown experience of successful disagreement and attachment without merger.

The imitative statements I used were not explanatory but expressive. They stated both sides of Francis' ambivalent "I need you . . . I hate you," without any effort to link or resolve them. The idea was gradually to expose and erode the intensity and unfamiliarity of such feelings, the way parents will tolerate young children who alternately kiss and poke them. Ideally, he would see me as a more or less helpful person, neither great nor altogether worthless. An ability to conduct his other relationships in the same spirit should follow. The distance between his boiling and freezing points would then increase, allowing him to experience the middle distance. It would be easier for him to be alone with someone.

One sign of success in this terrified Francis when he became aware of it. He had already discovered that in gaining intimacy he often felt swallowed up, but he had not known that he felt like doing the same to others. This was one reason why he frightened people away. He had a voracious yearning and expressed it with hungry looks. He began to realize that he was lunging at anyone who interested him. I associated this indication of cannibalism or orality with his failure to separate from his mother. His awareness of the behavior was an early sign that it was lessening. Francis went through a long period knowing that the only women who felt safe and drawn to him were those who did not interest him and thus stir his voracity. The most predatory aggressiveness lived up close to an innocent openness: eat and be eaten. I said, "When I want something, it runs away." Francis' wishes had to be spoken and validated; specifically, they had to be expressed passionately in order to be shared and spoken for him, then gradually reduced and made acceptable. This was the longest and hardest part of the work.

"I have no rights," I said for him. His mother had said, "Eat what's put in front of you," and Francis ascribed the same expectation to me. He was supposed to like the treatment, find good things in it, and do as he was told, despite its failing to make any difference at first and for a long time to come. My saying "I have no rights," he remarked later, seemed to say first that I was like him, and then that I wanted him to have rights. To have talked about his plight from outside would have left him alone inside. The patient without rights is like a prisoner who has no one in authority to whom he can protest, except for the very ones who have imprisoned him. Actually, family prisons are worse than real ones, because at least prison guards wear uniforms that identify them as such. Mother wears a "mother" uniform, and it is not until much later that one learns she is a guard. The therapist who talks about the patient's imprisonment is easily mistaken for another guard.

The ideal for Francis had been to turn the other cheek. In fact, once a hallucinatory voice had cried out those words and then told him to die. It is no wonder that people sometimes think they are Christ. Many have been told by their families (and have practiced through their role in the family) to sacrifice themselves. Profound goodness has the reward of saintliness, but at the price of death. Machiavelli, Marx, and Nietzsche all pointed to this exploitation of Christ. They warned that the good man is at the mercy of the exploiter and has to learn to drive the moneychangers out of the temple. I suspect that much religious teaching minimizes the danger because the temple may be controlled by the moneychangers, who naturally do not want to be driven out.

I did not say these things to Francis. It would only have been the case of one philosophy against another, and mine not the most acclaimed one. Worse yet, it would have been one more authority telling him what was right. Instead, I blamed myself for the slow treatment; in fact, *he* was paying *me*. It was my responsibility to construct the relationship in such a way that he had space in which to exist. My earnest statement, "I am responsible," was taken at first to be what he felt—Francis usually took responsibility for everything. Only gradually did it become apparent that the *I* was really *me,* that the treatment was *my* responsibility, and that at least here, in this space, he might be given something of his own.

Simple Empathic Statements

Empathic language helps, first, to find the other, gently and imitatively when the other is little present or vulnerable, more robustly when the patient is less easily frightened or distorted. The simplest form of this more aggressive empathic speech is directed at states of mind, which are expressed through impersonality and rhetoric.

Exclamations and Adjectives

Empathic exclamations are the range of short, emotional utterances by which the other's feeling state is acknowledged and shared. When we follow a person's narrative in an empathic way, we find ourselves automatically producing these exclamations. The narrative of a frightening experience causes feelings of fear in the empathic listener. Typically one exclaims, "How awful!" or "Frightening!" On the other hand, we may distance ourselves with such expressions as "Don't be afraid," "Why were you so afraid?" or "I wouldn't be scared of that." Note that the grammatical forms here are imperative, interrogative, and first-person declarative, not exclamatory.

It is easy to overstate the importance of words in these exchanges, since just as much is conveyed by tone of voice, gestures, facial expressions, and the like. Words are emphasized because they are the vehicles of expression most easily described and categorized. One can construct a small schema of empathic exclamations that goes from nonverbal utterances right up to the more complete empathic statements, which are termed translations.

The simplest empathic exclamations are the nonverbal utterances. It is amusing to recall the variety of clinical sounds one encounters in training and in oneself, but of course not all are empathic. Many psychotherapists learn early to make a small rising noise at the end of sentences, similar to the French "N'est-ce pas?" By doing so, they turn statements partly into questions, which is useful when one does not want to inquire directly. Harry Stack Sullivan described a method of changing the subject by using transitional noises of varying degrees of intensity.[1] So distinct are many such speech accents that one can sometimes identify a therapist's place of training by the types of noises he makes.

Empathic sounds are of many types and form an important supplement to what is usually considered the language of emotion, namely facial expression. Many different noises can be detected in the background of taped interviews with empathic therapists, conveying such responses as assent, protest, contentment, outrage, or sorrow. One reaction I noticed when patients wept: not only did I often feel like weeping myself, but I uttered brief, low cries. Darwin remarked that "crying out or wailing from distress is so regularly accompanied by the shedding of tears, that weeping and crying are synonymous terms." It is as if my moans had supplemented the emotional expression of the crying patient. Darwin also noted the striking contrast between the physiologies of distress and laughter.

> Why the sounds which a man utters when he is pleased have the peculiar reiterated character of laughter we do not know. Nevertheless, we can see that they would naturally be as different as possible from the screams or cries of distress, and as in the production of the latter, the expirations are prolonged and continuous, with the inspirations short and interrupted, so it might perhaps have been expected with the sounds uttered from joy, that the expirations would have

been short and broken, with the inspirations prolonged; and this is the case.[2]

New or unsympathetic students occasionally laugh when listening to very distressed patients. They are being antipathetic, that is, they have uttered the sound furthest removed from the patient's expression. It is also striking that such laughter is strongly resented by students who are sympathetic to the patient. Often the same contrast occurs within the patient, who laughs at the point of distress. Thus the individual establishes distance from himself by failing to empathize with himself.

Of course there are many degrees of empathy. Each of the foregoing utterances may be expressed with varying conviction, thereby placing the therapist at different degrees of closeness to the patient. Moreover, some feelings may be difficult to "get with." One example is contempt. I have occasionally been able to share contempt with a patient for some offensive act done to him and found myself making the "slight snort" that Darwin associated with the turning up and contraction of the nose and half smile, the sneer so characteristic of contempt.

Much is done in everyday clinical work with relatively indifferent sounds, for instance, variously toned "huhs" to indicate attention. This is a sort of minimal empathy; at least our attention is with the patient.

Adjectives of empathy, such as "awful" and "wonderful," comprise the smallest verbal step beyond empathic sounds. They provide a greater variety and precision than is available through sounds, but they tend to occur less spontaneously. So I tend to use adjectives or translational statements while attempting to get close to the patient, not when I am already there and responding spontaneously. Adjectival empathy, as it were, often misses its mark and must be corrected in keeping with the patient's response.

It is possible to take an empathic position between the active and passive attitudes. This is useful with secretly depressed people, the smiling depressives and hypomanics. The vital element is to be highly attuned. One must be intent, almost rapt, ready for the smallest hint of sadness, while simultaneously trying to absorb the whole person. At this point, I find that adjectival exclamations accompany the attention like punctuation marks.

Another form of empathic exclamations is accented adjectives, such as "How awful!" These are the spontaneous form of adjectival empathy and cannot be prescribed. Accented adjectives seem unctuous or patronizing when used deliberately, which sharply increases personal distance and stops the narrative flow. When occurring spontaneously, though, they express surprise as well as emotional attentiveness.

The reason the empathic stance exposes the therapist to surprise is that few can expect to share every feeling with equanimity. There are experienced people who never seem surprised because their knowledge of life has accustomed them to every emotion—but this is rare. Further, many therapists feel they should never express surprise, even in the presence of appalling clinical revelations. Whatever empathy they provide must, therefore, be carefully measured out lest unaccustomed feelings engage them.

While such exclamations as "Good God!" may introduce empathic statements and add emphasis—"Good God, that must be awful!"—more often they indicate difficulty in understanding, believing, or tolerating the experience described; the speaker pulls back from what has been recounted. As part of an empathic effort, such exclamations suggest a need for an affective reorientation in order to stay with the narrative: "Give me a moment to take that in." They call attention to the feelings of the therapist. These expressions can be included with a number of speech forms that are not intrinsically empathic but occur in the course of the empathic effort. Although not themselves empathic, they adjust the speaker, the hearer, or both, so that empathy is again possible.

Translations

A translation is the rendering of the patient's state of mind into words. The most succinct of these translations are many of the exclamations just discussed, such as "How wonderful!" "Terrible!" said with appropriate feeling. English does not have a comfortable structure that begins with the feeling state; we do not say "Terrifying is . . ." outside of poetry. Complete sentence translations generally make use of "It/there is . . .": "It is terrifying." An alternative would be a rhetorical question, "Isn't it terrifying?"

An important quality of these empathic translations is that they validate and do not attribute; they imply rather than ascribe the expressed state to the patient. For example, they would intimate "I feel terrified when I realize what you are experiencing," instead of stating "You feel terrified." This validates the other's emotions by accepting them as one's own. Curiously, this acceptance can be conveyed by the impersonal form, "It is . . ." This most personal of states is conveyed impersonally because it does not belong to any one person alone but might be participated in by anyone. We are saying it is natural, understandable, and shareable. The impersonality of empathic statements is illustrated even by those statements that use personal pronouns, as in "You must be terrified." The implication is impersonal: anyone would be terrified.

One definition of the impersonal is "not existing as a person." The dictionary states that the empathizing individual is infused with or participates in another's state of mind. The therapist's personality is momentarily replaced by or gives way to this state. To that extent he exists less as a separate person. Or, to use Carl Rogers' phrase, he becomes "a pane of glass."[3] Translations are impersonal in the special sense that they refer to states of mind seen as universal, or at least readily understandable. Furthermore, the two persons in the empathic experience are subordinated to the understandable state of mind. In part, the personal and individual give way to the impersonal and universal.

The second characteristic is that translations, like exclamations, exploit rhetoric, the art of expressive speech. Empathic exclamations and rhetorical questions are expressive forms, and declarative sentences, such as "That's awful," must be said expressively in order to do their empathic work.

It is hardly surprising that rhetoric should find its way into psychotherapeutic speech. I do not refer to a rhetoric that is aimed at persuasion, manipulation, or exploitation, although these are possibilities that psychotherapy and rhetoric share. The recommended uses of rhetoric are simply the uncovering and mastering of feelings through expression. Here we carry the old idea of catharsis a step forward.

Catharsis in psychotherapy was taken to mean the bringing of unconscious material to consciousness and permitting it emotional expression. It would thereby lose its power to create conflict. Difficulties sprang up from two directions. Often the patient's feelings could not be mobilized in the treatment, remaining stubbornly outside of it, perhaps outside the patient's life altogether. Second, and from the opposite direction, once the feelings were mobilized in treatment, sometimes they did not lose their power and pathogenic force. The patient could get stuck there.

The therapist's rhetoric, effective speech, addresses both of these problems. The activation of the patient's feelings is facilitated by the therapist's expressive force. Empathic language can, in many instances, offset the power of the resistances and direct the patient's material past them. This idea will be illustrated shortly, along with the suggestion that part of what has been called unconscious forces repressing awareness requires covert external reinforcement to be effective. When the therapist ceases to collude with the patient's resistances, perhaps by abandoning attitudes of coolness or excessive propriety, much appears that is new. It is as if the internal balance of forces is partly dependent on their external relations, much like the politics of modern nations.

The therapist's expressive speech assists in the opposite situation as well. To share means to divide or apportion. When we empathize, we reduce the patient's burden of feelings. When therapists remain aloof and unexpressive, they invite an escalation of the patient's own expressiveness, in order to convince or move the apparently unresponsive therapist. When, instead, the therapists share in the expressiveness, they demonstrate that they know.[4]

An Illustration

The following case illustrates these two contrasting features of simple empathic statements: the impersonal and the rhetorical or expressive. The difference between them seems to be critical, for they appear to balance and make each other possible. It will also be shown how empathic speech stimulates and deepens the narrative flow. Here is another test of successful empathy. Does the speaker stop or change the subject? Are the expressions of feeling increased or decreased? One of the moments of greatest clinical drama occurs when a strong empathic flow encounters a memory heretofore forbidden to consciousness or denied. Then we test the power of empathy against the resistances.

Gilbert, a thirty-five-year-old married man, was referred to me by his wife's therapist for help in "becoming independent." I was told that the couple had been very close and dependent upon each other through most of their ten-year marriage, but after therapy the wife took a job. Gilbert had reacted to this with "concern." He was a thin, affable man, quick and bright, but with a plainly deferential air. Surprisingly, he said that he was as eager for the referral as his wife had been to provide it. He claimed to have felt relieved by her growing independence and wanted to take steps of his own. He had in mind several artistic projects that had been postponed for years.

Gilbert's family experience had been difficult. His mother died when he was eight; his father left the care of household and son to the mother's sister. Gilbert said she was a wealthy, autocratic lady, who hated the father and was reclusive and preoccupied. As a result, the boy was largely cared for by servants, who remained his principal companions until he was sixteen. He remembered them as being friendly, helpful, and often protective against his aunt's demands. When he was twelve, his father remarried and tried to take the boy back, but the aunt stoutly resisted. The patient recalled not knowing where he wanted to go. He then found himself spending more time at his father's home, in spite of the fact that his father remained stiff and aloof. "I can't remember when he ever touched me," Gilbert said. It was reputed that the patient resembled his mother both in appearance and temperament. He had always been a lively, affectionate, and helpful child; however, his efforts to be close to his father seemed only to increase the older man's reserve.

The part of our work that I will present concerns an attempt to uncover the patient's feelings for his father. On one level this offered no difficulties; he was aware of his father's coldness, claimed to love him, and believed that his father returned the love in his extraordinarily reticent way. At the same time, he did not express any strong love or hate for the father. During the period of this first exchange, it was only possible to imagine the patient's deeper emotions; my spontaneous responses to him were as bland as he appeared himself to be. So I relied entirely on active empathic efforts in the exploration for deeper feelings.[5]

Gilbert: He never touched me. He would never even shake hands. [Said quietly and objectively, with more amusement than plaintiveness.]

Havens: It hurt. [Said off-handedly. The content of this message is affective, but the manner largely contradicts it. As a result, the therapist appears to be very much where the patient himself is, speaking so objectively of his father's coldness. At this point, if the therapist had been more expressive of the hurt, it might have provoked denial or argument. First the therapist has to put himself where the patient is; only then can he know what an acceptable movement away from that position might be.]

G: My stepmother criticized me openly. It was always a fight. Now we just don't talk. [In this early phase he regularly mentioned his stepmother or sister instead of expressing feelings toward his father. Women had often come between him and his father; in a sense the mother had, then the aunt, and most recently the stepmother. His sister had also been a factor because the father often was openly affectionate to the sister in the presence of the patient.]

H: It was infuriating. [Said with some intensity, matching the patient's. Women either had fought for him, as his aunt and wife had, or against him, like his stepmother and sister; there was little distance in his relationships with them.]

G: [Describes in detail several episodes, each of which involved his frustration by sister or stepmother. I was left wondering, "Where is the father?"]

H: The missing man.

G: My aunt took over, after my mother died. [Again, the mention of women following a comment about his father.]

This exchange could be termed "establishing an affective baseline." Several attempts were made, and all of them skirted two opposite dangers. On the one hand, the patient may adopt the feelings we assume he has, perhaps for safety's sake, thus misleading us. In contrast, if we are overly cautious in translating, we may reinforce any unfeeling or aloof image he has of us. It is like hunting: the hunter must make sufficient noise to flush the quarry, but not so much that he frightens it into paralysis or fresh concealment. What I sought here was the affective baseline, and it had two parts. One was an amused, slightly hurt, bittersweet resignation. The other was a quarrelsome, shrewish reaction, quick to occupy the ground of the first part if the resignation was disturbed.

In the second phase it was necessary to replace the bittersweet resignation with something more robust. The goal was to uncover or develop what I imagined were the "real" feelings of the patient. I say "uncover or develop" because it was unclear whether these feelings were already present in the patient, waiting to be uncovered, or would emerge as a product of creative interaction between us.

Note in the following conversation how objective elements, chiefly statements about states of mind, alternate and eventually mingle with expressive devices. The process resembles climbing, in that footholds or resting places alternate with bursts of activity, until the two unite in the excitement of arrival. We might also speak of an "emotional dialectic."

H: How much you must feel about him. [This represents a general forward movement but is said quietly. At this point I make no effort to express precisely what the patient feels beneath his resignation. I don't know and therefore have to explore.]

G: I felt he loved me. He just couldn't express it. [Now he stays with the subject of father and feelings, not replacing it with women.]

H: Perhaps it was frightening to him. [This is very objective. In fact it asks the patient to be objective about the father and to step into the father's state of mind. Essentially I am being empathic, but with the father.]

G: It's true he didn't have any men friends. [Patient complies, is objective.]

H: Oh God! [A simple exclamation of dismay—but not empathic because it expresses my state of mind and not the patient's. I use this exclamation to get his attention, in order to make a major empathic move. Note that the patient responds with a question. The usual sequence is reversed; the patient asks the question instead of the therapist.]

G: What do you mean?

H: He couldn't give even friendship, and you must have wanted love.

G: I wanted him to touch me. [Starts to tear. The patient is now both objective (descriptive) and expressive; fact and feeling are being brought together.]

H: At least. [This occurs spontaneously; patient and therapist are now close enough for passive empathic efforts to suffice.]

G: I always wanted him to hold me.

H: To be loved, and to love him too. [The first is said more matter-of-factly than the second, which has a rising cadence. The patient still finds it easier to acknowledge his desire to love than his wish to be loved. But both these phrases refer to states of mind, simply translated and expressed in an atmosphere of feeling.]

To recapitulate, an affective baseline had been established and then some feelings were uncovered or developed. The alternation and combination of objective, descriptive states of mind and expressive or rhetorical statements may be critical to this process. Objective statements such as "anyone would feel . . ." validate the patient's state of mind, and the speaker appears to understand intellectually. In addition, statements must be made expressively, or the speaker will have appeared not to understand in the emotional sense. He will seem to be an exception to his own rule. Perhaps the validating and expressive statements must be first divided because two separate defenses are being overcome: repression of meaning and isolation of affect.

The third and final phase illustrates the collisions mentioned earlier: the further development of feelings and staying with the patient in the face of considerable resistance. This stage may result in the type of bond that is formed between people who endure difficulties together, as in military service, sports, and some marriages. Note in this exchange how resistance moves from the patient's historical and contemporary experience directly into the transference. Also note how I do not attempt to minimize the resistance by fully merging with the patient. In my last two remarks, I do express part of the patient's state of mind. However, by using the pronoun "you," I attribute rather than fully empathize. Either I was instinctively asking the patient to take responsibility for his feelings, or I was afraid to share emotions I myself may resist.

G: I made this birthday present for him. It wasn't much. I mean, I made it in school carpentry class.

H: Still, it may have felt like a labor of love. [Itself a little labored.]

G: I remember wrapping it and writing "Pop," a name he didn't like.

H: "Love to Pop."

G: My stepmother was nice, for once. She knew how hurt I was. [A woman again appears in place of the father feelings.]

H: She may have known how much you loved him. [Emphasis on the "how much," making the statement expressive. I do not try to circumvent the woman but use her as a bridge in the empathic statement to return to the father feelings.]

G: I handed it to him and he put it down without unwrapping it. He did the same thing at Christmas. [Again the lighthearted, almost flippant tone. The patient is collecting instances of past and present rejections to prove the futility of his loving. Soon this resistance also appears in the transference.]

H: You must have been terribly hurt. [The patient immediately touches the outer corner of his eye, as people often do when they sense tears.]

G: He never liked us to cry. [Noticeably looking away, so that his eyes can't be seen: the resistance in the transference.]

H: I remember your saying once, "How easy it should be to love him." [Again the expressive emphasis on "how easy," making this almost hortatory.]

G: But it was so hard . . . [crying].

H: And you love him so much. [I also feel like crying.]

G: I would say the Lord's Prayer at night and think of him and cry.

H: If only he could be your loving dad!

Every vital development of language is a development of feeling as well.

T. S. ELIOT

Complex Empathic Statements

I have suggested that imitative and simple empathic speech can either express our emotional response to the other or be used to reach something unexpressed in the other. These, however, stand helpless before the great mass of complex and contradictory feelings that are present in most cases. At times there may be no understanding. At others it may be necessary to celebrate the naturalness of what is felt, against the patient's need to deny a feeling. Or there may be many conflicting states to understand. The material that follows suggests three bridging phrases that help to deal with these situations. Each has the impersonal and exclamatory elements found in empathic translations, and also something more.

Let me say at once, and again, that mastery of language alone does not constitute empathy. A therapist's disinterest, inattentiveness, or lack of ability to contain the other's feelings can alter the effectiveness of even the most appropriate language. On the other hand, a powerful empathic ability can redeem language that is otherwise prying or even critical. Above all, these phrases are not to be taken as formulas, restricting the freedom of therapists. I am describing the means by which a therapist attunes himself to some of his patients. As I have stressed, one needs to place oneself attentively near the other, to be alert to expressions of feelings, not to concentrate on the verbal content alone.[1] At first no particular feelings or appropriate verbal expressions may come to mind. Then a variety of static-like fragments will arise, some seemingly unconnected to the patient, others interpretive or reflective, until we catch sounds or phrases rising to our lips that suggest feeling states of the other. The means, quite marvelously, follow upon the intent.

"No one understands"

Ostensibly, "No one understands" translates a feeling of being misunderstood or abandoned. But the statement contains a systematic ambiguity that allows it to be still more serviceable. It suggests that both "I" and "no one" understands: "I understand that no one understands." As a result, "no one" statements stand in relation to other empathic statements as scouts do to the main body of soldiers. Both reconnoiter unknown territory.

Suppose that we mean to empathize with someone whose combination of background, appearance, and personality offers no easy point of empathic contact. If such a person does not feel understood, we can certainly comprehend it, since we ourselves do not understand. At this point in the relationship, a shared "no understanding" is the only point of contact. "No one" statements are therefore preliminary empathic statements.

"No one" also postpones stating who has not understood. The patient may feel awkward complaining that particular persons do not understand. Furthermore, "No one understands" creates a tension between the state of mind projected and the world to which the phrase "no one" points. Instead of keeping exclusive attention on the mental state of not being understood, it points to the wider world where someone who does understand may be. The tension created will equal the resentment against "no one" from the person who has the feeling state. For this reason, such statements should be made in expectation of a later, franker externalization. The speaker must be prepared for the patient's discovering, perhaps suddenly, who that "no one" is. While the negative may not be a part of the unconscious functioning, as Freud asserted, it is a profound impetus to interpersonal functioning. Perhaps because opposition is built so deeply into our evolutionary equipment, the statement "No one understands" invites the reflection "Someone should have understood" and also "So-and-so did understand." It opens territories of memory to be jointly visited; it is history taking.

"No wonder"

"No wonder you were frightened!" is a statement that celebrates the naturalness of feeling. As in the earlier example of "You must have been frightened," the personal pronoun "you" is depersonalized by the implication that anyone would have been frightened. But something fresh appears in addition to the exclamatory and impersonal elements—contributed by "wonder." While "no one" reconnoiters the field of blame, "no wonder" clears it. This is an active use of empathy, not only a sharing of feeling but a justification of it. The speaker places himself between the emotion and whatever precipitated it, connecting the two. He implies, "In view of what happened, it is natural to be frightened."

The celebration or justification is achieved by positioning oneself at the point of denial. The connection between event and feeling has perhaps been only dimly conscious or denied. There is a theoretical empty space between event and feeling, created by a pushing apart of the two. The event appears to be severed from the feeling because the person involved cannot believe that those responsible for the event would have done such a fearful thing. To maintain a secure image of the person involved, emotion and incident are separated.

This pushing apart is characteristic of denial and different from the pushing down of feeling, event, or both feeling and memory that is characteristic of repression. This explains why the event and feeling in denial are "known" but their connection unknown.[2]

It is now possible to grasp the importance of the word "wonder." Patients may recall having "wondered" about the unexpected behavior of persons dear to them or those they depend on. For instance, "Why is mother doing that?" Mother's behavior was puzzling, a source of wonderment. As long as this confusion remains, the actions will be denied; the event causing the wonderment is disconnected from the ordinary conception of a parent. As a result, the parent and the feelings precipitated by the incident are kept apart. Breaking down the denial means breaking in on the wonderment.

"No wonder" is therefore a denial of a denial: it was *no* wonder. Because the patient's denial is actively maintained and defended by a need to preserve the old image of the offending persons, denial of the denial may only temporarily fill the space between event and feeling; they will soon be pushed apart again. Permanently breaking down the denial depends on frequent reiteration of the "no wonder" and a change in the patient's conception of the offending persons.

In time, "It is natural" will replace "No wonder." By regularly placing oneself at the point of separation, event and feeling are repeatedly joined until they are seen in relationship to one another and reconnected. The power of repetition to rejoin, however, is not due to the repetition alone; nor does it come from the increased awareness of the connection. Reconnection is a function of something else, namely, the empathic experience. A time has finally arrived when the patient has not had to face the unacceptable alone. Introducing the state of wonder to the patient who has wondered, and still wonders, places the therapist where the patient is. Later, when referring to events they have denied, patients often remark that the denial would have been unnecessary if there had been someone with whom they could have shared and reviewed the events. The empathic experience provides that someone.

"God forbid/knows"

Because so much of human suffering springs from conflict, being with the patient means being with opposing impulses or demands. It is not enough to locate the separate conflicting elements; this may only increase the pain by bringing the conflict to clearer consciousness. The empathy of conflicting states includes sharing the pain of conflict itself. Bridging statements and efforts do this.

Edward, twenty-one years old, was literally carried into my office by distressed parents who seemed barely able to carry themselves. They said their son did nothing but stand in the kitchen and drive knives into the breadboard, once in a while saying "shit." Actually, none of this behavior was new; what had provoked the parents was something the mother had done. She placed her hand on the breadboard and told him to stop: he just missed her thumb.

This case was remarkably similar to one Sullivan described many years ago.[3] Like Sullivan's patient, this young man was puzzled by his own behavior and had nothing but kind, albeit unenthusiastic things to say about his parents. His mother in particular had been his closest friend and adviser. In both cases the technical problem was transparent: how to bridge the gap between the patient's ostensible loyalty and gratitude to the parents and his threatening behavior.

My patient and Sullivan's had both been closely cared for, extensively warned about the dangers of the world, and actively prevented from learning the social skills that most people acquire without thought. Sports were dangerous, dancing and cards sinful, and driving a car could lead to accidents. In short, almost everyone was up to no good; the only safe place was home. At the same time, my patient wanted to be an athlete, he liked to watch dancing, and his supreme ambition was to own a car. These goals were not apparent until much later, though, because Edward presented himself as content and normal, if a little puzzled by the excitement he had caused. One looked in vain for a twinkle in his eye, a bit of a bootlegger's wink—some recognition that he had managed simultaneously to terrify the perfect parents while preserving his apparent love of them. I concluded that this was no game at all, but a deadly contest of wills; he was fighting for his soul and self.

Such a contest is difficult to enter successfully because the patient himself has had to play a double game. He knows that he is cared for; he is identified with his protectors, who as a rule are also identified with him. Any attack on them, either by himself or others, is therefore an attack on him—hence his puzzlement about his destructive behavior. He is not conscious of being rebellious or even feeling anger, although such patients often are aware of being fearful. The revolt is manifest only in his occasional actions. This is what is meant by "dissociated behavior."

The conflict is seemingly inaccessible because there is no self in the patient with whom the conflict can be discussed. The patient is unaware of being in conflict. His occasional behavior expresses his indignation, while his usual behavior and his speech express the very viewpoint he is indignant about. His conscious, apparently responsible self cannot even admit that the occasional behavior is his own; it is crazy. This is the socially acceptable way of denying responsibility for a part of himself. Furthermore, he can get many professional people to agree that the occasional aberrations were due to a sick brain, and no more his responsibility than the measles.

If attention is called to his hostile wishes, they are immediately denied or disowned. If his fear of the parents and his subjection to them is noted, it is just as quickly denied. Even if remarks are made about the difficulty of his situation, the constriction of his comfort, or, more forcibly, the price exacted for all the parental security, the comments fall on the patient's deaf ears. The official position is that everything is just fine.

This is the point at which psychotherapy of the most serious conditions stops, if it can be said to have begun. It is therefore "no wonder" that all sorts of measures, surgical, electrical, or chemical, are used to quell what is looked upon as a crazy revolt.

Sometimes it seems that the patient is being killed with kindness or, more accurately, has never been allowed to live. The usual parental task of fostering independence has been replaced by an encouragement of dependence. This may be caused by one or both parents having an intense need to keep the child close. The need may originate from the loss of an earlier child or from the belief of one or both parents that they know how others should behave. It is necessary to add that no one is sure how much the

deeply imprisoned person *evokes* these qualities from parents, turning otherwise unremarkable parents into know-it-all tyrants. There
are individuals who bring out the worst in others.

The challenge of such deeply imprisoned people to psychotherapy can be termed a problem of acknowledgment. The dictionary states that *acknowledge* means "to own or admit knowledge,"
implying that what is acknowledged is genuine and that any material previously presented is less than genuine. The imprisoned
person's rage is at once a genuine expression of his rebellion and
an expression that is disowned or unacknowledged by the rest of
his personality. The patient does not "arrange" his behavior so
that he can be both angry and innocent at the same time; he is
genuinely surprised and appalled by what he has done. There are
two genuine and opposing claims that will not make room for
one another, and there is no bridging person.

In contrast, when the hysterical patient both wishes and forbids
the wish, there is an element of self-deception or bad faith that
allows the conflicting elements to remain in the same personality.
As Freud wrote, the patient both knows and does not know.[4] It
is this half-awareness of each side of the conflict that allows the
therapist a relatively easy access. The half-awareness signifies a
capacity for integrated function with which an alliance can be
formed.

When the therapist tries to reach the imprisoned person, he
must first realize that there is no representative body to contact.
He is like the foreign neighbor of a country at civil war. In essence,
it is necessary for the therapist to bring into being a provisional
government with which he can deal. Bridging statements are the
verbal materials for establishing it. The seat of governance is found
in an unexpected place: the patient's reaction to his own behavior.
It is the very incomprehensibility of his behavior, the fact that
the patient terrifies himself, that allows a point of contact. The
experience of meeting a self that is crazy shakes the preexistent
self, opening the way for a new solution.

The therapist is able to enter the state of civil war because he
naturalizes or validates the patient's apparently bizarre behavior.
This introduces the warring parties to one another. The intro-

duction is possible because the conservative part of the patient does not want to acknowledge its craziness. So it welcomes a view of the rebellious element that naturalizes it, just as a sick man may welcome being told he has a specific, treatable physical disorder. The danger of accepting a specific disorder is that the patient is left inwardly divided.

Earlier I said that the psychotic character is didactically useful in clarifying general processes of change. The psychotic recovery presents, in gross terms, the same processes that are critical to favorable change in many less devastating conditions: a person must first be found or created to resolve the issues at the heart of a free existence. It would be convenient if "no wonder" statements could achieve the necessary integration. Unfortunately, "No wonder you say 'shit' and stab the breadboard—you want to escape" would meet either fresh incomprehension or silence. The patient has not yet acknowledged that he wants to escape. It is the wish to escape, and the difficulty of doing so, that must first be established.

The pressure against acknowledging the wish to escape comes from the identification with the parents, dependency on them and fear of their disapproval. These are the usual tools of imprisonment, and formidable tools they are, even though they are not usually applied with the ostensible purpose of imprisonment. They may actually be applied with the stated intent of liberating or at least saving. For this reason, the person's right to be free is not usually at issue, however much it is covertly undone. Just as the patient's horror at his own psychotic behavior makes possible the first alliance with him, so the generally accepted ideal of his being a free and developing spirit serves as the beginning point for offsetting the parents' complete authority.[5] Once again, it should not be concluded that the parents are the villains; the patient may have instigated much of his imprisonment. For this reason, therapists and psychopharmacologists need to beware, lest they too be lured into making the patient dependent and imprisoned.

In the cases where the therapist secures a historical review, it is relatively easy to highlight the combination of protection and incapacity that has been fostered. At that point, an acknowledgment of the wish to escape, despite the good-hearted efforts made to protect the patient, is quickly made. Further, the step toward validating the patient's awkward efforts at protest is not difficult to take. In time, the empathic "You must have wanted to protest" or "No wonder you say 'shit' " suffices.

The difficult cases are those in which no historical review is forthcoming. These can be recognized in hospitals and clinics, if the individuals have been admitted before, by the lack of meaningful historical detail in their charts, even after prolonged hospitalizations. There has not been enough of a person present to give, or even have, a history. In such instances, the work of establishing a provisional government falls entirely on the therapist.

The prototypic form of the effective language is "God knows" or "God forbid." The material of the provisional government is brought to the patient with comments that represent both the imprisoning agency and the independent wishes that are imprisoned. "God knows you must want to escape" often directly represents the patient's delusion that there is a great power watching and controlling. What the statement introduces is a possible union of the conflicting elements. In a state of extreme ambivalence, the conflicting elements have lain about like scattered puzzle pieces. The bridging statement begins to bring together the separated parts.

"God knows you must want to escape" should be said at first descriptively, matter-of-factly. A delusion that is partly fact is being repeated. This connects the therapist with the patient's thought process. The connection can be made still closer if the bridging statement is done imitatively: "God knows I must want to escape." The provisional government remains largely helpless, though, until the wish to escape is connected with the frightening behavior. The naturalization of the frightening behavior is begun by repeating the bridging statement with a new emphasis: "God knows you must *want* to escape." The statement is no longer purely descriptive. The wish to escape and, still faintly, the right to protest are shared. The power of the comment is increased by an ambiguity that appears in the first part of the sentence. "God knows" at once repeats the parental authority *and* lends support and emphasis to the wish. Here is a beginning of the subtle loosening of the parental authority. A different god is being introduced, one who might wish the patient to escape.

By changing from "God knows" to "God forbid you should want to escape," we can illustrate the tidal or dialectic process of that escape. "Forbid" suggests that a person should not want to escape, implying a forbidding god. However, the bridging statement is gradually rendered at first a little, then more strongly, sarcastically. The therapist comes to stand with the patient in his wish to escape, even to defy the authorities. At this point, often well into therapy, the provisional government is no longer provisional. A swinging back and forth between one part of the conflict and the other prevents either side from paralyzing the slow movement forward.

In summary, these statements voice the patient's dilemma. "God knows and forbids" invokes the parents who know and forbid. But, when the therapist says "God knows you must want to dance," he states two opposite positions at once: mother does know, and therefore it is dangerous; but at the same time, a different god knows that everyone wants and needs to dance. The impossibility and the dangerousness of the patient's position are acknowledged by the therapist saying he knows that the parents know and forbid. Simultaneously, the patient is beckoned to a different set of values and to the validation of his wishes. The double statement moves closer to what will be identified later as performative: it defends the patient against the forbidding, internalized, and also external parents.

Like Sullivan's, my patient's first experience was relief. Edward began to see that he had understandable wishes that were being frustrated and that his behavior made sense; he no longer felt so odd. He would not have felt relief if the war between himself and the parents had been exacerbated; he probably would have become even more psychotic. Because both points of view had been acknowledged, no further action either of rebellion or submission was demanded.

The first order of business with a new patient is to acknowledge that his behavior may serve sensible ends. However misguided or even dangerous the patient's behavior appears, it may express, at least partially, intentions with which anyone is able to identify. The principle recalls the legal presumption of innocence until guilt is proven.[6] It is a remarkable principle. I have seen many symptoms melt away with acknowledgment.

What seems especially remarkable is that the melting away often occurs before the patients' wishes have been fulfilled. This suggests that some of the symptoms may be a result of unacknowledged conflict as opposed to conflictual desires, and that the unacknowledged conflict undermines the sense of self. This does not mean that Edward's saying "shit" and plunging the knife into the breadboard, and nearly into his mother's thumb, was not the expression of a wish. His confusion and puzzlement, however, along with his feeling crazy, were not the result of his frustrated desires, which were still unfulfilled after the acknowledgment. Instead, they may well have originated from his inability to admit and contain the conflict.

In short, these bridging statements appear to be effective precisely because they make it possible to acknowledge the conflict, which is the first step toward integration. Voicing either side alone would only provoke the condemnation of the other; bridging statements are "equal time." Furthermore, each side is expressed with feeling, rhetorically and empathically, and the intensity of the feeling on each side is shared. Finally, the very intensity, given with equal force to opposing sides, expresses the pain of the conflict and relieves the patient of some of that pain. It could be said that a simple, direct statement of the conflicting elements would bring what previously has been denied to the patient: making it known. Unfortunately, this knowledge cannot be sustained, and the conflict kept conscious, until the pain of the contending elements is borne and a person is brought into being capable of the bearing.

A Hard Case

I want to strengthen the concept of bridging statements by extending their use to another mental state that has defied psychological resolution: the hypomanic character. The hypomanic person burns with excitement and rushes into the future, all the while seeming to fend off difficulties and defeats. He has not integrated sadness with courage, elation with reality, past with future. He needs to assume the complex, bittersweet attitude ·that is central to wisdom, being able to say "Enjoy it while it lasts" during prosperity and "This too will pass" with the onset of adversity. These are the means by which human beings balance experience.

The hypomanic person stimulates our amusement, even laughter. Inexperienced observers can be expected to smile, and even old hands may have to settle themselves in for work. Attempts to stay with either the excitement or the sadness are generally frustrated. Allowing ourselves to become excited, for example, by joining or admiring the patient, stimulates him, but this emotional transmission does not result in staying together; typically, the patient moves away. Sometimes regarded as the central dynamic of elation, intense closeness can be experienced as death.[7] Staying with the patient's sadness is also difficult. Sad events are denied; the patient immediately changes the subject or becomes annoyed. Only the gravest clinical manner, and the most persistent mention of events, will permit more than transient contact with hypomanic sadness.

The requisite language will express the patient's yearning to be admired at the same time that his bankruptcy is acknowledged. This seems inconceivable at first glance. Even "no wonder" statements, ordinarily so useful when dealing with denial, fail us. "No wonder you speak of love and adoration, there is so little of it" only exposes that, in fact, it is a wonder. The hypomanic individual has not only separated mood and fact, but has reversed the mood anticipated for these facts. The "no wonder" comment, so appropriate when he feels miserable, fails to be empathic when he is not. It *is* a wonder that he can feel high when so much is low.

It is also remarkable how the empathic attitude generates its own solution. If it *is* a wonder, then we can express that, using "wonder" and not "no wonder." The hypomanic person asks to be an object of wonderment; to be empathic requires doing just that. Paradoxically, the therapist's capacity for wonderment will continue to grow, once an acknowledgment is made of how much the patient has had to deny.

The operative word is courage: the capacity to preserve one's spirit in the presence of danger and despair. It is the admiring acknowledgment of courage that bridges elation and despair, allowing us to hold the patient in a positive relationship, while at the same time exploring his situation and feelings. "How have you been able to hold your head so high, when everything has fallen apart around you?" Note that this is a rhetorical question. It does not invite an answer, but simply expresses both admiration for the courage and an understandable fear of the facts. Again, the empathic statement is both exclamatory and impersonal.

The courage that the patient displays is easy to admire. Hopefulness and putting up a good front are virtues to nearly everyone but psychiatrists. Yet, at the very moment of admiration, the cover is removed. It is striking how quickly admiration for the defense opens the door to despair. Indeed, the careful worker must not go through that door too quickly but should hold back a little in shared congratulation of the hopefulness. Ideally, the patient will then push us toward the sad facts, in review of which, God knows, courage will be needed afresh.

I have said that "no wonder" statements are the denial of a denial. Conversely, the statements that bridge hypomania and depression reverse a reversal or, in more formal language, correct a reaction formation. Once again, discordant elements are bridged, and the movement toward integration begins.

*Imagination is the power of the mind
over the possibility of things.*

WALLACE STEVENS

Extensions

While translations and bridging statements are meant to put us within the other's experience, extensions permit movement through that experience. The state of mind "It has been difficult" is extended in time with "It has been difficult for a long time," or in space with "It is not only difficult at work but at home." Adverbial modifiers such as "for a long time" make it possible for the therapist to place himself at particular points in the other's experience. This can be termed an exploration of another's world. Plainly, many statements applied to that world will not fit. The patient may respond, "No, only at work. Home was different." We can relocate ourselves and once again be with the other. Of course there are hazards; we are not reconnoitering now, as with "No one understands." We are exploring, even invading, the experience of the other.

Sounding the Limits

Such an exploration is especially critical in the presence of suicidal intent. It is important to know if there is any time free of that intent; if, for example, there is any future except death. Through extensions, it is possible to probe the farthest reaches of the sui-

67

cidal wish, noting if the patient follows—which can be called "going below" or "sounding the limits." "There is no future except death" bespeaks the patient's extremity and, accepted by the patient, tells the therapist where the patient is. Still, the patient may not follow.

P: I did want to die.
H: It may still be what you want.
P: I don't know.
H: The pain continues.
P: I feel so terrible.
H: It may not be possible to imagine any time free of it.
P: I thought if I died it would stop.
H: That might be the only time.
P: No, now I feel I will be better. [The patient's mood lightens, and she goes on to discuss several positive aspects of her world.]

This illustrates an emphatic exploration of another's point of view along the dimension of time; it exposes both despair and hope. It does not indicate what would have been more frightening, the view of endless continuity: "It may not be possible to imagine any time free of it." Or stopped time: "That might be the only time." Each of these extensions of despair were expressed for her, but she declined them. What is important here is that the exploration was made empathically instead of interrogatively, representing the state of despair more directly than most questions could do. The empathic exploration enables the therapist to share the extent of despair the patient feels. In contrast, questions tend to encourage the subject-object distance, which may be dangerous when the patient already suffers alone in extreme despair.

What follows is a more complex example to help show the variety of categories of inner experience.[1] In this case it is primarily the experience of internalized (introjected) others in time, but it also includes extensions in drive, feeling, and spatial states. Note the contrasts of real and perceived time, and of real and introjected persons.

P: I was waiting for my mother to understand.

H: Perhaps she never will. [A painful extension into the future.]

P: Even when she's better than she used to be I don't expect it. [Declines the future extension for the real mother, but confirms it for the introject.]

H: You kept waiting and hoping. [Returns to the past experience of the introject.]

P: I think of her always the way she was. There would be months on end when I would wait. [Confirms the eternal changelessness of the introject; at the same time, perceives and examines it.]

H: Waiting and hoping, and needing too. [An extension along the lines of drive and feeling.]

P: That seemed the slowest time of my life.

H: What's the old saying, "A watched pot never boils"? [Although rather awkwardly used, the proverb is quoted to demonstrate sharing of the painful distortion of time brought about by helplessness and impatience.]

P: I watched and watched . . . I needed her so much. I'd often sit in the kitchen [the proverb was also an inadvertent spatial extension], then she did come through and it seemed too late.

H: Sometimes there is here, too, the same waiting and hoping. [A spatial extension to the treatment situation, both in the objective space of the treatment room and in the subjective space of the transference.]

P: You seem to have all the time in the world.

H: Will I ever boil? [Taking in at once the mother, kitchen, the treatment situation, and a possible double meaning.]

P: I suppose you mean cooking, or getting angry. I don't know.

H: You probably didn't know then either. [A temporal return.]

This example goes beyond the implication with which this chapter began, that extensions are primarily exploratory. Here extensions are being used to move the patient through time and among objects. The more aggressive language utilizes frankly ascriptive pronouns: "Perhaps she never will," "You probably didn't know then either." It is no longer a simple sharing.

Locating

The search for unintegrated feelings in the body—Semrad called it "tour of the body"[2]—naturally takes a spatial form: "You must have felt it in your heart," "Perhaps it moves," "There were feelings in your genitals." The following exchange occurred between me and a fifty-four-year-old woman who had recently experienced her first recognition of genital sensations, with the conviction that she must be going mad.

H: Perhaps it began in your stomach.
P: Somewhere there. I hardly noticed.
H: Then it moved farther down.
P: I didn't know what it was, except that I was terribly embarrassed.
H: There hadn't been many feelings there before.
P: I didn't remember any. Now I thought I was going mad.
H: There were these feelings in your genitals.
P: I was terribly embarrassed.
H: They didn't seem to come from you.
P: I kept blanking out.
H: Maybe it was love?
P: I thought of that, but it seemed dirty.

One purpose of my remarks was to avoid talking about sexual wishes as opposed to the experiencing of their bodily location. Working with the categories of particular time and space helps prevent the abstraction of experience, which the use of even such a familiar concept as "wish" entails.

Many people describe having trouble with getting themselves "together" upon awaking from sleep. There is a carryover of scattered images and feelings from dreams or a sense of dislocation that may even include body parts, for example, when the limbs do not seem so much a part of the body as usual. One patient told me that throughout his adult life it had taken a full hour to collect himself into a coherent experience of bodyhood upon awakening. His feet or arms would seem disconnected, unresponsive to command; not asleep in the familiar sense but at a greater distance than usual. With the sense of disconnection was a sense of being himself scattered about, hardly there, unable to muster an act of will. This man was also separated, even when walking about, from much of the rest of his spatial environment. He frequently got lost and was unable to remember the names or appearances of streets where he had lived for many years. These phenomena dated from a long period in an orphanage after the breakup of his family home.

Extensions are invaluable to this process of locating experience. For example, memories of home can be explored for feelings, particularly with the help of temporal extensions: "There were many times when it must have felt different there." As a rule, much lies ready to be shared, but there are closets, bathrooms, and perhaps the parents' bedroom, in the revisiting of which unintegrated feelings will be met. Some patients will not need the help of extensions; if allowed to, they will unfold on their own oedipal preoccupations, the primal scene, and castration anxieties. However, for those many instances in which the patients cannot spontaneously verbalize their experience, or do so only after a long period of time, temporal and spatial extensions provide a structure for remembering.

Approximating

Extensions are useful not only in traversing time and space—they also have a use in approximating the elements of conflict that the spatial term "approximates" itself suggests. During the recovery of schizophrenic patients, a reduction in the experienced distance from hallucinated objects and a change from angry or flat to depressive affect can sometimes be observed.[3] This is in keeping with the internalizing process associated with depression; with the onset of depression, the hallucinated objects come to be experienced within the schizophrenic person's body. We can speak of an approximation of psychic parts or, quite literally, a gain in self-possession. Sometimes the hallucinated objects even become friendly and advisory, or are absorbed altogether into the everyday experience of conscience. This we can call an integration or reconciliation of psychic parts.

The following example will illustrate how extension statements can facilitate this process of approximation and integration. Essentially, it demonstrates how concrete spatial and temporal language can serve not only to locate the patient's experience, but also to help move it.

Mildred, a forty-five-year-old woman, had been repeatedly hospitalized for assaultiveness associated with ideas of persecution. She had lost contact with her family, left her job as a secretary in a Washington political organization, and led an increasingly isolated and vagrant life. As is characteristic of many paranoid people, she retained her pride and sparkle, and was contemptuous of other patients encountered in treatment facilities.

In the course of the initial interview, it was possible to connect her idea of being pursued by a murderer, part of an ill-defined plot, to an incident that preceded her first hospitalization. While employed by the national committee office of a political party, Mildred uncovered a scandal involving a prominent figure. In her characteristic stiff, outraged fashion, she disclosed the details to a number of persons, only to find herself increasingly isolated in the office. She resigned soon afterward. Although she wanted to tell what she knew to some authority, she was unable to find anyone she trusted. She grew fearful that her knowledge of the secret put her at risk, and she also felt a conflict between her outrage at the incident and her loyalty to the party.

It was easy to compare this secret and its resulting conflict in her adult life with a similar course of events in her childhood. Mildred was the youngest child of parents who had divorced when she was four. The mother then worked as a governess for wealthy families, among which the patient grew up. She partly identified with these families and was sometimes openly ashamed of her poorer sisters and father. She stumbled upon a scandal there too—a liaison between her mother and one of the employers—and revealed the facts to the mistress of the house. The mother was discharged, and the patient placed in an orphanage. The two had never discussed any part of this episode.

Mildred left the orphanage as a teenager and worked hard to get secretarial training, taking great pride in the clothes she could now afford. She felt considerable jealousy from her still poor sisters, and she snubbed their large families and lower-class husbands. The oldest of these sisters had been kind to her when she was in the orphanage, and the patient revered her. It was a crushing blow when this particular sister would not take her home after the first hospitalization. Mildred said she felt murdered.

Note the sequence here of childhood conflict, the adult precipitating event that partly recapitulates the earlier conflict, and the psychotic ideas that appear to generalize to the world at large. This progression is not unfamiliar or surprising; it is the bread and butter of those who study psychoses and families. What needs to be stressed is the technical difficulty of approximating the three elements: childhood events, adult precipitants, and delusions.

As a rule, if the therapist can successfully "translate" the delusions into the precipitating events and then into the childhood conflict, patients stop expressing the delusions. Instead, they talk about the precipitating and childhood events. This is the most convincing reason for believing that the delusions express those events, announce or bespeak them. Note that Mildred also explains why the events cannot be addressed directly. Not only may the childhood incidents be denied or repressed, but, as important, she fears that those who are listening may not believe them or may even blame her. She may get herself into deeper trouble by openness, as she did with the political party and the mistress of the home in which her mother was governess. This patient's experiences of confiding in therapists were no better. One doctor insisted the childhood events were fantasies, earlier versions of her "delusions." Another doctor, noticing the patient's bitterness toward the oldest sister, asked Mildred what she had done to alienate her.

It is interesting to observe how little will remain unconscious when given a genuinely receptive climate. Such a climate depends on the ability to translate and approximate the different elements. The patient cannot be left alone to do it. The connections are painful; the conflict between her outrage and her loyalty is apparent. Further, she cannot know in advance what the reception of the therapist will be. By empathically approximating the elements himself, the therapist both shares the pain of conflict and indicates his willingness to believe in her experience.

Nothing could make this work more difficult for the therapist than the conviction he must reassure or correct. Such impulses will be irresistible if the therapist feels that normal people are "secure" and the fear of murder, for example, is largely pathological. In any event, reassurances of this kind are becoming harder to provide in a time of random violence, horrific accidents, and the threat of nuclear disaster.

Note in the following conversation how I took the initiative at the start of each exchange, the first being concerned with the Washington situation. Also notice, as with my opening remark, that many of the interventions are not exclusively empathic; they present hypotheses about external events (and therefore belong among the projective and counterprojective statements to be discussed shortly).

Havens: But you may have really stumbled upon something certain people didn't want anybody to know.

Mildred: Mmmm . . . that's what I think happened, that I stumbled on some information that happened to be true, but that I myself didn't know that it was true. This is what I thought.

H: That might have been one of the reasons you wrote the letters.

M: Yeah, I wrote them to General X because he was with the Committee and he took the letters and turned them over to the FBI. Well, the FBI was part of the whole plot.

H: Well, you certainly didn't expect him to do that.

M: I didn't expect him to that. It was a very stupid thing for him to do.

H: You in fact wonder whether he was part of the funny business going on.

M: I think it was more ignorance on his part, Doctor. [The extension is stopped short.]

H: Well, he certainly seemed to have been a very loyal person. [I retreat.]

M: He was very loyal to the Committee. He was running down in Washington, and I had a meeting with his secretary to see how much I actually knew was going on. Yeah, and the minute they found that out, they probably covered me anywhere I went, and I didn't know I was being covered.

H: That must have been a terrifying experience.

M: Well, it was.

H: Because to think you were in possession of something that people were so frightened of anyone knowing, that they would want to take your life.

M: I said to myself so many times since then, Doctor Havens, is your name . . . ?

H: Havens . . .

M: Yeah. I said to myself many times afterwards that if there wasn't any truth in what I wrote in those letters, why didn't they just come to me and say, "Why look, you're a sick girl, you have to leave here and not work here anymore." But they didn't do that.

H: Why didn't they deal directly . . . ? [An imitative statement that she finishes.]

M: . . . as if I were really sick then?

H: Yeah, why did they go over to the FBI?

M: That's what I mean, an . . .

H: Well, that certainly increased your . . . [I have arrived where she is, so we complete each other's sentences.]

M: That increased my wanderings, and my philosophy that I had stumbled on the truth.[5]

But moving offered no security:

H: Because you still have possession of this information. It still isn't clear what to make of it, right?

M: Well, once I go around acting as if all has been forgiven . . . I have done this for periods of time in my life . . . like acted as if I did dream the whole thing up. [She offers me the opportunity to dismiss her whole concern as fantasy or delusion.]

H: Yes, but that's no solution because you don't know that . . . there's no way of really being sure.

H: Well, that's right.

M: So that indeed, you still may be fingered by somebody who might be afraid of what you suspected, or are suspecting.

H: Yeah, right.

M: So that this shadow has never been lifted from your life.

Then a movement into the more distant past, out of which the patient selects her relationship with her sisters, and particularly the unjust treatment she felt she had received from her oldest sister. Note the beginning approximation of the paranoid fears to her feelings about this sister.

H: You know, the terrible injustice of you, who had good things when you were small, and your mother would not have to slave the way she did, and then your sisters got out of it in time . . . right? [After the breakup of the family.]

M: Yeah, but they married laborers and they had a lot of problems, and then, when I got a little older, I was associating with a lot of people that had a great deal, and I had nice clothes because when I got out of school I was determined that the one thing I would have was nice clothes, and you know . . . because for years I had gone with shabby clothes. And my sisters became jealous and spiteful in view of all this . . . and they . . . in other words, my eldest sister, who was my favorite sister, which was the shock of it all, she was the favorite one . . . and yet she threw me in an insane asylum and she was going to leave me there forever.

H: She threw you in an insane asylum?

M: She was gonna leave me there forever. She wrote me after I had been in there four months . . . I wrote to her and said, "My doctor says I can come home." She never answered the letter. Well, they came about three o'clock in the afternoon on Christmas Day and they told me that they couldn't afford the gasoline going to and from the hospital and I had maybe sixty dollars in the bank, so I had to pay for the gasoline.

H: You mean you were stuck in this insane asylum?

M: Yeah, and I had to pay for the gasoline for them to go to and from their houses.

H: You're joking?

M: No, I'm not joking.

H: That's incredible, isn't it?

M: Isn't that incredible? And then when I got out of the hospital finally, there was so much complaining about the cost of food and I was occupying this shabby . . .

H: Well, you were a proud person, so it was a very humiliating situation.

M: I was occupying this shabby room and I didn't have transportation to and from the city and I had a terrible, terrible time that first time I went to the hospital and, or, the second time I went to the hospital I had a terrible, terrible time, and uh . . . so I finally worked my way out of the hospital by taking a job on the outside and getting out that way.

H: It sounds like even back there, there was this attitude toward you that was perilous, really.

M: This spiteful attitude, because when my sister slammed the door on the insane asylum, she looked satisfied. She had this satisfied look on her face. Yeah, and I said to myself, "I'll never put myself in her hands again."

H: Yeah, be sure you don't, right?

M: Because she . . .

H: Because you can't trust her . . .

M: I can't trust her, and so after I'd been in the hospital, she wrote and she said, "My husband and the boys don't want me to have anything further to do with you . . ." In other words, I wasn't . . .

H: She wrote that in a letter?

M: Yeah, and I was trembling and I gave the letter to my doctor, and I was trembling, and he said, "What are you shaking for?" and I said, "This is the letter . . ."

H: "What are you shaking for?!" What if somebody had said that to him!

M: Yeah, well he didn't know what was troubling me . . . so I gave him the letter and I let him read it, and he read it and he said, "What have you done to your sister?" And I said, "Nothing."

The paranoid person's world is entered into, understood on its own terms and shared. Then the scattered elements can be approximated, when they lie apart, or separated, when they have been condensed, so that an integrated person can gradually be formed.

Causal Extensions

Clinicians new to therapeutic work are always asking "Why?" Patients are then being asked to testify about themselves, often against themselves. It is a curious situation; the psychiatric patient is asked to explain his condition to his helper, a reversal of the usual medical role. This may be because psychiatry and psychology are young, and in our ignorance we ask for help.

Causal extensions offer a partial escape because thereby the task of inquiry is shared. If I say "Why didn't you call?" I am judgmental, inquisitive, and assume that the patient knows. On the other hand, if I say "You must have had some good reason for not calling," I put myself with the patient and extend that empathy investigatively. "It is easy to see why you might not call" does some of the work of "No wonder" and at the same time throws open the inquiry. Causal extensions assume an understandable, human (never-to-be-fully understood) reason for the behavior, and begins its discovery with the patient.

Causal extensions can be made for their own sake, for insight, or simply because feelings attach to ideas, and these feelings may need to be shared. Psychiatric explanations and hypotheses are seldom far from the patients' minds and are just as seldom comfortably held. In the current interpretative climate of much psychotherapeutic work, patients sit waiting for the next insight with their fists clenched. Small wonder, for it is rarely good news. As a result, to enter the contemporary patient's mind is to enter into an uneasy relationship with ideas, indeed, with many of the same ideas that therapists have.

Equally or more upsetting are the concepts patients develop in the course of becoming sick. When dissociated material breaks into consciousness, people think they are going mad. Because of the special attitudes people have about mental illness, they do not usually rush off to the doctor; more often they increase their secrecy and vigilance. This means they are feeling, "It is not acceptable to go crazy," and by extension, "The cause of mental illness is something to be ashamed of." Consequently, in my view therapists do well not to ask about causes, for fear of increasing that shame. The empathic statement, "It was more than a person could bear," at once extends our investigation into the unbearable and shares the pain.

Being able to share what another heavily bears lightens that load; at the same time, it indicates where the bearer is and what that existence consists of. We now move farther out into the social context of personal existence and the language that can help to manage the forces at work there.

Interpersonal Language

Master, I marvel how the fishes live in the sea . . . Why, as men do a-land—the great ones eat up the little ones.

Pericles

Good Management

We continue to speak to the problems of human isolation and domination that express themselves as characterological or situational difficulties. In general, and with much overlapping of function, empathic speech addresses isolation while interpersonal speech addresses the many forms of domination.

If finding another means to be taken into another's world, can it not also mean to be "taken in"? Isn't the very openness to the experience of the other an invitation to the actor and the impostor? In these instances the tables are turned. The actor and impostor wish to impose their imagined worlds on ours; it is no longer simply a matter of our seeking to find them. The problem of finding another then becomes a problem of power, invasiveness, and the management of personal distance.

The verbal instrument for the management of distance is interpersonal language. With it, invasive patients can be deflected. Patients' expectations and imaginings of invasion can be reduced. The therapist's own utterances can be put in such a way that patients feel free to take them or leave them.

Finding a Working Distance

Psychotherapists cannot work if the patient's mind is outside the room. They also cannot work if the patient's mind has invaded theirs. I first realized this when a depressed patient depressed me to the point of my feeling hopeless about the case.[1] I needed more distance on the suffering.

Mental invasiveness is both real and imagined. Not only do some minds alter and shape others; it is possible to imagine them doing so, often with the same result. Many people cannot sit quietly in another's presence without imagining themselves being criticized by the other for their silence. Without any overt evidence of attack, they feel attacked. One patient confided that he always felt either deserted or impinged upon and could seldom recall being alone *with* anyone. Occasionally he got this feeling while reading with his wife in the evening, though often he felt impelled to ask if she was annoyed with him for not talking. Once, fishing with a friend in his boyhood, he had felt comfortable with another person, but that was long ago.

Winnicott suggests that the capacity to be alone with someone develops from the experience of being alone with the mother; the child's immaturity and dependence are balanced by the mother's support. Of equal importance is her being present without making demands: she lets the child alone. People who cannot be alone, either by themselves or with another, may not have had this noninvasive experience. The problem of invasiveness, real and imagined, can therefore be called the problem of learning to be alone with someone. The adult who invades or cannot manage others' invasions, or who imagines unreal ones, must recapitulate the child's experience of first learning to be alone with someone. The therapist's task is threefold: he must distance himself from any actual invasiveness of the patient; he must refrain from reinforcing any expectation the patient has of invasiveness; and he must offset the patient's imaginings.

The state of being alone together can be termed a working distance. Each party respects the other's space. Therapists accustomed to working close and moving in with their feelings and ideas may crowd some patients, in order to promote rebellion or obedience. Other therapists are themselves poorly protected and will need to back off from invasive patients. It is a matter of not attending so avidly, of drawing back psychologically. Very polite people have difficulty with this: they have never learned to hang up the phone.

The language of empathy moves the therapist into the patient's space. This is noninvasive if the empathy is accurate, if it is the patient's feelings that are experienced, not the therapist's. Accurate empathy is, again, of particular significance in achieving a noninvasive closeness in which the patient has someone present on his own terms. It is not the quintessential experience, however, because empathy aims at merger or identification rather than a working distance. The full experience of noninvasive closeness awaits the development of a capacity to stand undistorted near those who shine forth fully on their own.

Balancing Power

It is systematically difficult to know how much people differ in their power. This is because the seemingly most powerful person must manifest that power through someone, so that the willingness or eagerness to be enslaved or overpowered is itself a power. It has been effectively argued that slaves possess their masters, both by their masters' dependence on them and, more subtly, by the corruption that power causes in its possessors. The absence of resistance in one personality encourages many other personalities to expansion, as if nature's abhorrence of a vacuum extended to mental life. This seems most evident in politics, but it is suggested by the experience of family life as well. Authority and obedience appear to condition one another to the point that natures perhaps not inherently tyrannical can become domestic Hitlers. The same processes affect psychotherapy.

It should not be concluded that every underdog designs his own enslavement, overlooking the fact that powers do in fact differ, that some personalities are difficult for even well-integrated people to resist. I recall hearing my father and his middle-aged friends describe meeting Douglas MacArthur. They were not great admirers of the general; the meeting occurred because he was seeking political support. My father said that after speaking half an hour with MacArthur there wasn't a man in the room who would not have gone to the window and jumped out if the general requested it. Such power is a critical part of successful generalship, when heroic acts must be requested and obtained. Yet these skeptical men were surprised to find themselves so entranced.

Charisma is the word most commonly used to describe such power. The pomp of office, a striking appearance, and a historical reputation contribute to it. But there have been personalities devoid of any office, reputation, or even appearance who have been able to exert a startling influence, and many of them have been psychopathic. The clinical study of psychopathy suggests that these individuals exert their influence in three ways: by will, by not creating doubt or anxiety, and by shrewdness. If the psychotherapeutic patient is psychopathic, understanding these mechanisms is necessary. Yet, because the same mechanisms shape many human interactions in less dramatic ways, therapists must always be prepared for them, in many contexts.

In these contexts, the term "will" means willfulness and determination, a will that is not pliable or easily turned aside. The charismatic will generates excitement, the wish to please, even passion. The subject initially feels the presence of someone exciting, then begins to feel the excitement in himself. This is an active or invasive empathy that may sweep through crowds and even entire nations. The charismatic will is also certain; it does not tolerate hesitation, skepticism, or anxious doubts. However, the usual or "normal" human will is, if nothing else, doubting. Uncertain of his powers, the usual person tends to suspect the uncertainty of all ventures, the role of chance and fate, and the rich possibilities of mishaps and the unexpected. This everyday skepticism approaches cynicism among the noncharismatic and is expressed in Murphy's law: if something can go wrong, it will. It is far removed from the buoyant optimism of vaunted leadership, which is often represented as the ideal.

Nevertheless, such optimism, kindled by an eager patient and susceptible therapist, can invade psychotherapy, creating the expectation that the therapist *knows*. This turns doubt into something sick or obsessional and perhaps makes the patient feel responsible for his own destiny, whatever the history of circumstances or mishaps. Of course, the charismatic therapist will be delighted to propagate such ideas, but even modest workers must have tools to offset the hopes many patients have about the therapist's miraculous powers. If they do not, therapists will carry a great power of seeming to know. Patients, in turn, will try to guess what pleases the therapist in order to elicit the secret wisdom, vainly waiting in the hope of being told. Therapy can be indefinitely prolonged when the therapist seems to defend a secret knowing that the patient hopes to unlock.

Shrewdness is the feature of charismatic leadership which is least often described. The charismatic leader must know which strings to pull. He must identify the gullible and pacify the doubters. Some learn early on the streets, unprotected by parents or caretakers. Some become outright psychopaths, able to deceive with a dexterity, if not a breadth of purpose, that would rival Napoleon's. There have been shrewd, handsome bank thieves who take a piece of brown paper, scrawl on it the name of a mythical bank, a large sum of money, and someone else's signature, then cash it. The average person often cannot cash a check at his own bank because he exudes guilt and doubt. The successful thief radiates confidence, even serenity; he feels entitled. Moreover, he looks over two or three banks before he finds the suitable teller. She must be young, unattractive, new to the world; no one should have flattered her before. Maybe her hair has been freshly done, so she has hopes. Then he makes his move. The goal is to engage her in easy conversation, gently flatter. Above all, she must do as she is told, never look at the old piece of brown paper. Of course if she does, he will have an amusing story, and nothing will come of his "mistake."

Excitement, confidence, shrewdness: the trick is done. Either patient or therapist may fall victim to it, and even where strong charisma and psychopathy are not at work, lesser degrees of the same qualities may empower patient or therapist. Further, the obedient, overeager patient may ignite in therapists charismatic skills they did not dream of having. This is especially true where a therapeutic relationship is supported institutionally, as with hospitalized patients or those who are part of training programs. Here the conviction of supporting the institutional truth may empower therapists, and a fearful eagerness to conform may enslave the patient. Such conditioning processes are not easy to detect; the therapist can also reward a measure of disagreement or independence which is then entered into for the purpose of pleasing the therapist in a further way.

It is not enough to say that psychotherapy depends on respect, even appreciation, and that the therapist extends himself so he will know when the patient's sickness leads to psychological predation or slavery. It is not enough because predation and slavery are statements of power that cannot be offset by reason and argument alone. A central contention of this book is that power can only be opposed powerfully, meaning that the therapist must have power and use it. Empathy may be necessary to find the patient, but then the patient may need to be defended against overpowering forces—or patient and therapist may need to be defended against one another.

Clearing the Field

Freud wrote about holding back and paying attention:

> The technique, however, is a very simple one. As we shall see, it rejects the use of any special expedient (even that of taking notes). It consists simply in not directing one's notice to anything in particular and in maintaining the same 'evenly-suspended attention' (as I have called it) in the face of all that one hears. In this way we spare ourselves a strain on our attention which could not in any case be kept up for several hours daily, and we avoid a danger which is inseparable from the exercise of deliberate attention. For as soon as anyone deliberately concentrates his attention to a certain degree, he begins to select from the material before him; one point will be fixed in his mind with particular clearness and some other will be correspondingly disregarded, and in making this selection he will be following his expec-

tations or inclinations. This, however, is precisely what must not be done. In making this selection, if he follows his expectations he is in danger of never finding anything but what he already knows; and if he follows his inclinations he will certainly falsify what he may perceive. It must not be forgotten that the things one hears are for the most part things whose meaning is only recognized later on.[2]

It was Alfred Margulies who first pointed to the curious symmetry of empathic and interpersonal language.[3] He showed that each clears the clinical field but from the opposite directions of, respectively, therapist and patient. The fundamental rule of empathic work—to clear the therapist's mind of prejudgments, diagnoses, and ideas of all kinds and to experience the patient simply as he or she appears—means to open the field to a fresh experience of the patient by the therapist. The fundamental rule of interpersonal work is the opposite: everything the patient presents is to be seen as a fiction, an artifact of the social world, and needs to be offset. In this case the clinical field is cleared from the direction of the patient; he should have a fresh experience of the therapist.

Working distance expresses the idea that the patient needs to be brought within range or, in the opposite case, extricated from too close an engagement. Balance of power expresses the related idea that neither patient nor therapist should overwhelm the other and that human interactions fall readily into patterns of predation and slavery. Clearing the field expresses still another related conception: that psychological cognition, the determination of psychological facts, is very difficult; it is easily contaminated by either therapist or patient.

The observations of psychopathology largely elude quantification. This means that small indications of psychopathological phenomena may be mistaken for the sick state itself. The problem is obvious in the delineation of affects where, for example, a minor blunting or isolating of affects may be mistaken for schizophrenic flatness. It also occurs in the description of verbal phenomena. Dissociated speech may be infrequent. But is there a dissociated state? The same can be said about catatonic phenomena. In their full-blown form, bizarre stereotypical gestures are unmistakable.

Yet everyday life is replete with slight, occasional, self-conscious peculiarities of gesture. Are these merely tics and signs of nervousness, or are they indications of latent schizophrenia? As a rule, one must wait and see. The point is that the absence of clear-cut numerical markers among psychopathological phenomena can result in overdiagnosis, the too-easy ascription of patienthood.

Psychological cognition is also contaminated from the patient's side. We can seldom determine to what extent patients' self-presentation is a function of their reaction to us. Sullivan says that therapists should learn what their typical impact is on the clinical situation, surely a wise idea. Yet even a sophisticated knowledge of such effects will not ensure freedom from distortion. The patient is probably unique. The therapist does not know his particular effect on this person, so that what is fact and what is artifact must be carefully studied. Even the multiplication of observers does not of itself yield objectivity, since each of the fresh observers may be imposing a similar distortion.

One would like to know two things: does the psychopathological phenomenon have more than a transient existence within the life of this particular person, and is what we observe a function of the social field? We cannot assume the transience, stability, or dominance of this social field. Before reliable observations are made, most clinical situations can be described from either the individual or the external points of view; witness the debates of analysts and social psychologists.

It is characteristic of the psychoanalytic method that keeping open and not concluding should be accomplished by the diffusion of attention that Freud described: nothing in particular is to be noted. In existential work, the tendency of expectations and inclinations to lead to conclusions is combatted by the "psychological-phenomenological reduction," the accepting of phenomena for what they are, the idea that they have no latent content. Whereas a discipline of attention, especially of listening, is at the center of psychoanalysis, an attitude of openness or credulity toward phenomena is central to existential work. Curiously, both avoid concluding by opposite routes—skeptical in the case of psychoanalysis and credulous in the existential situation.

The interpersonal attitude avoids concluding by still another, even more skeptical means. The interpersonal therapist believes that the credulous attitude toward phenomena may leave the observer shaped or invaded, because the phenomena could push him to conclude. He is also skeptical that the psychoanalytic observer can "hover," since he fears that the forces at work will reach up and shape that observer. The interpersonal viewpoint implies an immersion in phenomena not unlike the existential one. The interpersonal worker, however, is eager to put down fresh phenomena as well as to receive the ones he is given, lest the given ones carry the day.

In other words, to clear the clinical field, therapists must cultivate attitudes sharply opposed to one another. Empathy is credulity operationalized: the goal is to be "taken in" and in the process to locate another. Interpersonal statements are skepticism operationalized: the idea is not to be taken in, not to allow the patient to settle assumptions or projections upon the therapist. The approach is fictive. The clinical phenomena encountered are assumed to be products of the interaction, imaginary creations of the moment, parts in the patient's and therapist's personal dramas. The issue of enduring personal individuality is put aside. Say that the therapist is doing this to the patient—would he be different if the therapist were different? Here the therapist does not want to be regarded as a particular figure, just as he does not want in empathic work to conclude prematurely that he has met the patient based on his recognizing the patient as tall or male. The fictive is investigated by unsettling assumptions that the patient makes about the therapist; the impact of the social field is measured by unsettling it.

This unsettling utilizes the random; the therapist's random statements help to keep things open. Unfortunately, this application of the word "random" is similar to that of "free" in free association; both are relative and partly undefined. "Random" should be elucidated as it is in the dictionary: "lacking a definite plan, purpose, or pattern." Nevertheless, our psychological experiences and theroies indicate that such a lack of aim or guidance may only be apparent. All sorts of influences, including counter-transferences, actively guide even the freest or most random associations. It is a paradox of analytic theorizing that one of the most deterministic of psychologies should even speak of free association. Of course, analytic theorists mean that free association is free from secondary process, from active, conscious efforts at organization or censorship. From what aim, direction, or guidance are projective statements free? For example, is this randomness the rule of free association transferred to the therapist?

If we could answer these questions in a satisfactory or even consistent way, there would still remain the vexing issue of application. Is every conclusion or provisional stopping point to be shaken, challenged, and an opposite datum suggested? It is true that the same question can be put to Freud's recommendation. Is the analyst never to focus his attention or reach a conclusion? Surely interpretations, especially those of resistances, require such a focusing, and they of course are also suggested.

Common sense dictates that Freud's recommendations be taken in a less constricted spirit. There are different tasks for the analyst at different times. The avoidance of focused attention is a central guide, but it would be ridiculous to apply it to every moment or situation. If the patient stops paying his bill long enough or endangers the work in some other way, there will clearly be indications for paying a great deal of attention. This is the spirit in which the random should be applied. It is an opening up of the clinical field promoted by the diffusion of the analyst's attention and the use of random statements. The diffusion of attention prevents the analyst from prematurely closing up the field. Random statements also keep the field open by counteracting the tendency of the patient to conclude prematurely in his turn. In addition, such statements help the therapist to see other possibilities.

My first efforts at not concluding led to an oppositional stance. If a patient decided that something was X, I would suggest it was Y. Then it occurred to me that random remarks were less oppositional and therefore less argumentative. The point was to respond freely, not just in disagreement. Free response depended less on a diffusion of the therapist's attention than on what can be called a lightening of attention. I allowed my attention to wander; what I encountered in that wandering or random looking was also to be held lightly. The operative expression was, "It occurred to me."

This creates a discourse by possibilities. The close comparison is to projective testing, in which the unfamiliarity of the stimuli, even in the Rorschach of their not "making sense," seeks in the patient an equal freedom for revelation. This revelation is one purpose of the random remarks and, as will be seen, the freedom of the therapist's speech is a generous payment for the patient's freedom. Yet the power for revelation is not the main function of interpersonal comments. The main function is to open fresh possibilities of human existence. To this end, the random in psychotherapy has the same central role that evolutionary theory gives it in the struggle for natural existence. The random, in the form of chance mutations and genetic groupings, offers to all creatures the possibility for new strategies in the battle for existence. Most of these changes may be worthless or destructive, but their occurrence is thought to be perhaps the only means by which life escapes the heedless repetition of old patterns in situations where they are no longer adaptive. It has been suggested that human creativity is also partially a function of random capacities of the higher human brain.[4] The very ability to make errors and to take unfamiliar paths liberates humans into the new and sometimes the constructive. It is conceivable that the random has an identical role in psychotherapy.

Happily, the psychotherapeutic random does not have to be built into the germ plasm to be effective. Possibilities can be mentioned, considered, and dismissed with the same freedom in which they were conceived. The idea is to open the struggle for human existence to fresh lines of thought.

Empathic and interpersonal methods respectively test for individual and field effects. Each method is available to rescue the patient in a clinical field dominated by social forces, or to dissolve any premature individual description or objectification. This is what is meant by clearing the clinical field.

Being Alone Together

A patient of mine seemed distracted during one session; plainly his mind was elsewhere. I knew he was in love with his secretary, who happened to be on vacation, and that he felt uneasy about his love. It was raining that day in Massachusetts, so I said, "I hope the weather is better in Jamaica." He was startled, as people are when someone appears suddenly beside them. We then spent a long time with the secretary, starting in Jamaica.

The patient had been distant. I did not want to drag him from his beloved and so I joined them. Perhaps I decreased the distance separating the patient from me too abruptly, since he seemed startled. But he was not offended. Conversations are wisely started with remarks concerning the weather—the original Rorschach cards in which we see what we want. I had hoped the weather was better in Jamaica; I had not wished her ill. He could feel that I was on his side as well as beside him, and hopefully a working distance had been attained. It is necessary to avoid dragging around or overwhelming the mind, which needs space.

A first clinical question should be, "Does the patient move toward us or away?" Of course some people are quiet and at a happy distance. Most patients, however, are frightened, eager, or both. They move away from or toward us, and at times oscillate between the two. Many can be categorized in an instant; you can almost feel them leave. Their eyes become vacant or distracted, the voice fades, and the content of speech is disconnected. Customarily, eyes and voices reveal more than faces and bodily movement. Other patients are obviously approaching, perhaps with the eyes yearning or angry and the voice eager. The therapist feels crowded.

There are many minds that are separated from one another by a highly tremulous and refractive medium. Meeting under such conditions is like reaching for an object under water, where the slightest movement of the hand may deflect it. The "water medium" intimately connects the two minds because disturbances are so rapidly transmitted. Moreover, the medium is refractive: the object does not lie in the direct path of vision but at some angle to it, so that it cannot be reached in a straightforward manner.

Whether we speak of being alone together or seeking a comfortable distance or a more stable medium, the important fact is the mental propensity to retreat in some cases and to impinge and be impinged on in others. If the patient is rushing forward, we need to step aside in order to reduce mental presence. To do this, I become a little scattered or absent myself, forcing the patient to stop and look around to find me. If I said "Slow down and take it easy" or "Why are you coming on so strong?" it could be interpreted as commanding or critical, and thus precipitate a debate before a working area had been established where such discussions are useful.

Some patients never slow down and look around; they continue talking whether or not anyone is listening. It is the high sign of clinical narcissism, when a patient does not have enough interest or sensitivity for others to note their absence. This self-absorption can seldom be usefully addressed. An unusual action would be more successful, perhaps an overly extended cough or making a slightly disturbing noise. Will the self-centered person notice? One can calibrate the degree of narcissism by the amount of disruption necessary to catch the patient's attention.

The goal is not to escape, however desirable that seems. The object is the establishment of a working distance, and to accomplish this both parties must acknowledge and respect the presence of the other. A gentle nudge may ease the oblivious person into sensing the existence of another person, without perceiving it as a threat. It is most important to avoid reinforcement of oblivious behavior, or conveying the idea that the purpose of therapy is to encourage indifference to others. If I do reinforce indifference, I can only blame myself if the patient is furious when I interpret what I have encouraged.

Gently shaken, the patient may look around to observe what

is happening and notice me momentarily as a separate person, not simply the fascinated ear he had imagined. Then I can briefly and respectfully say hello, fully realizing he will resume ignoring me after the signal has been received. I do not expect more, since this is as much of another human being as he can manage right now. It is only necessary that the contact be comfortable, brief, and deferential. Possibly the patient requires immense distance from others because previous experiences have left him emotionally allergic to people. Cultivating his tolerance and decreasing the space can only be accomplished gradually.

This, then, is a form of interpersonal management. It is not obviously empathic because the distances employed are so great; and the posture of judging another, and deciding what should be done with him, is alien to joining and sharing. Nevertheless, the management of distance also makes empathy possible. We cannot be empathic if we are overrun or feel patronized, and it is difficult to be understanding of someone we cannot locate. Moreover, empathic work is itself a means of controlling space. Assuming the viewpoint of the patient makes the most radical reduction of distance possible. The same empathic work sometimes extricates the therapist from being a target for the invasive patient, for the therapist has joined him in his resentment of the world. Let us turn now to the various forms of language that help to establish a good working distance.

> *[Every gesture] has to be thoroughly rehearsed, in order to present an image of relaxed spontaneity.*
>
> HENRI MATISSE

Projective Statements

The simplest form of interpersonal speech is the projective statement, which is a making of marks and remarks. Projective statements are declarative sentences that evoke.[1]

"It was a nice day in August."
"No, it was raining, I remember mother said it would clear."
"Then your sister got mad."
"She said mother was crazy."

A mark has been placed and the patient is stimulated to add, correct, or erase. The whole picture can be built with such marks and remarks. There are similarities to the style of painting Cézanne pioneered. Form was not built with outlines but with dabs of color. Each dab evoked and changed the color values of the others; the structure of the painting emerged from these colorful fragments. Cézanne said he wanted to paint the entire picture at once because each part changed every other part, and the meaning of any segment could only be discovered in the whole.

Listen on the bus or subway. People make empathic exclamations, ask questions, and listen in silence to reveries and associations; yet perhaps the most powerful engine of verbal intercourse is the statement of fact or possibility. It is comparable to the use of percussion in chest medicine. The physician places one finger on the chest wall and strikes it with the middle finger of the other hand. The note resounding signifies the degree of density beneath. In this way physicians can outline heart sizes, tumor masses, and levels of fluid accumulation. Prior to radiographs, this was often the only method available. Statements of fact or possibility operate similarly. Note in the following exchange with my patient Will the variety of depth, detail, and agreeableness of these resoundings.

Will: She never seemed sad. Daisy did, except in her letters.

Havens: Maybe then she could remember more.

W: I like writing and receiving letters. Pam wrote about getting settled now, knowing what she wanted, and she said she was getting over her fear of machines. [This fear had obstructed their three-year relationship. They had planned to build a house together, but she became afraid of the trucks and the chain saws.]

H: In some ways Daisy and Pam seem opposite, one excited, the other steady and shy, but in their letters, they each seem to change.

W: Daisy gets sad. Pam is articulate. Otherwise she seems too shy to talk. Her boyfriend lives near me. He knows exactly what he wants—a musician.

H: Perhaps a lot like Daisy's Peter?

W: No, Peter's spacey. [A nice clean erasure.]

H: Well, she could have made him that way, crawling all over him. [Earlier the patient commented that he had recently seen Daisy and she had been overattentive. He had attempted to reciprocate but was embarrassed. Later he had written to her about it and asked how she could have acted this way when she was involved with Peter.]

W: She wrote she'd met this boy I knew in college who said I was brilliant, could be a great architect.

H: Maybe why she was all over you.

W: She often said I gave off an aura of strength. Other people in her family said that too. I wish I'd brought those lousy corners to show you. [He is attending a woodworking class and claims to be unable to form good corner connections.]

H: I guess I wouldn't be marveling at your strength then.

W: [laughs] They're terrible. [He is resounding to a shared pleasure in his clumsiness. He seems to feel we both can enjoy it.] I've begun to dream about doing something else. It always seems to happen this way. One month into something and I wonder why I do it.

H: Better to dream now and not be stuck with something you hate later. [I feel the patient may be setting a trap by inviting a typical fatherly response: "Stick with it, you'll never succeed unless you buckle down," etc.]

W: There's a guy at school who does perfect joints. I asked someone how come. He said "That guy sacrifices his personality for his joints." [The critical, perfectionist father ideal could easily settle on the therapist. Have I successfully removed enough of it for the patient to speak this way?]

H: That sounds like your father. [He sacrificed his personality and family for business and politics.] Can one do something well without being like him? [Hopefully an imitative statement.]

Left to associate, this man was largely silent. Questions tended to make him defensive and elusive, perhaps because his father was a keen interrogator. It was also true that empathy softened him to the point of dissolving; he wallowed. On the other hand, he worked well "outside," when dealing with concrete details and possibilities set down for his perusal, in keeping with his woodworking and architectural interests.

Also note that Will's responses were not pedestrian or simply factual. The most dramatic was the shift while describing his "aura of strength." Suddenly he wanted to reveal his failure, which was so evidently in contrast to the fellow student's success. That shift underlines a subtle development up to this point, which would be even more noticeable if the whole interview were before us. Apparently his two girlfriends, with whom he reported having failed relationships, remained very much interested in him. One was even attempting to remedy a fear that had impeded their relationship, and the other was, puzzlingly, "all over him." Both were eager and revealing correspondents. He was describing his strength and appeal; at the end he suggested a reason for undermining them. Success would have made him like his classmate or father, who in this patient's view had flawed personalities.

It would be misleading to suggest that the marks put down reflected any overall strategy. Indeed, such a plan, unless it were loosely and unobtrusively held, could only terminate the free exchange; one wants to avoid any air of ponderousness or even direction. Certainly the therapist's prejudices and stupidities will be obvious enough in any free exchange.

I am aware that nothing could seem less professional. Yet medicine begins with the routes of access nature gives us, and only later are pictures taken of the brain at a distance. Freud understood this—he expected the analyst to hear a pound or even a ton of static for every ounce of the unconscious. The point is to set the other in motion as naturally and richly as possible. It is not surprising that this should be accomplished through a means of conversation to which everyone is accustomed.

The Power of Detail

It is also no accident that this making of marks is a familiar means of conversation. Projective statements evoke, in part, through the power of detail.

When I ask "What was the weather like?" I give and request a level of abstraction that invites still more abstraction. Inwardly, the respondent adds other questions to the first one, such as "Does he mean temperature, humidity, or barometric pressure?" or "Do I remember accurately?" The apparently simple question can become a nightmare of schoolrooms and examination books that summon up accuracy, intellection, thoroughness. Contrast the first statement with "It was raining on Sunday." The patient may respond, "No, the sun was shining." He does not have to think about the abstraction, weather. Rain fails to fit his memory because he may recall the sun. It is easier for him to remember because he is not wondering what the other wants. Moreover, since he operates on a level of concrete detail, feelings are mobilized that carry with them memories and trains of associations. Such is the power of poetic language, which is supremely concrete.

The smell of almonds evoked Proust's world. Is this because deeper, more emotional, less abstract and refined levels of mind are reached by sensory details? It is impressive that one does not have to be right to evoke: mention of rain is at the same time mention of a class of events, weather; memory of the actual event lies not far away. It is like multiple-choice questions, which jog the memory. Rain did not fit and something else was demanded.

Napoleon said that God is in the details. He meant that for lack of a nail the shoe was lost, then the horse, followed by the message, and the whole battle. His greatness as a general was not only in the boldness of his conceptions, but also in the mastery of detail by which he rendered the conceptions real. No one was less patient with ideas he could not see in the world. General Grant is another example. Sherman wondered if Grant thought at all because everything seemed to appear to him as concrete details that were each a call to action.[2]

It is interesting that successful warfare and poetry should both stand in such dependence on detail. Possibly it is because conceptions, however grand, do not move as in war or move us as in poetry unless they are concretely realized. War and poetry are matters of movement, which is accomplished in solid steps.

Psychotherapy, unless it is to be an intellectual exercise or an abstract discussion, also depends on movement. This applies not only to a general sense of personal change or development, as opposed to stagnation or repetition, but to the very process of psychotherapy. Therapists and patients experience a feeling of emotional movement, at its most intense, of *being moved,* complete with its verbal or cognitive aspects, including a flow of memory, contact, creativity, and imagination. This does not mean that there are no useful occasions of summing up, reviewing, and even formulating, in which the movement stops and an account of it is given. Certainly some personalities seem to need more of this than others. Yet, even when this is done for such clarifying purposes, therapists often arrest the movement at their peril. This is especially true when the patient's life has had little movement.

Making marks and remarks is a powerful engine of psychotherapeutic change, partly because of its evocative power of detail. There is another source of evocativeness that can be termed the hypothetical, which implies a willingness to be wrong.

The Hypothetical

Therapists carry, in varying degrees, the burden of authority. It is usually because of some presumed authority or at least superior knowledge or experience that they are consulted. In much medical and some psychological work, the burden of authority is carried happily. A discrete lesion is suspected, tests are made, and the treatment prescribed. Compliance is the patient's role, not only because the tests and experiments may be painful and time-consuming but also because the patient is essentially ignorant. The more medicine becomes dependent on complex technologies, the more this is true; physicians grow progressively less reliant on what patients report.

In much psychological and some medical work, this relationship between authority and ignorance is reversed. The psychotherapist almost entirely relies on what the patient communicates. Moreover, the meaning of what the patient relates is largely dependent on his further productions and the unfolding of the patient-therapist relationship, to which both parties contribute. Finally, the results of these exchanges gain much of their significance from the decisions that the patient makes as to what he wishes for himself. Here of course he can look to the authority of the therapist, who in turn must be careful that the patient's search for freedom does not fall under a fresh domination.

There will be many psychotherapists for whom this description of their work will be unrecognizable. Many behaviorists, some cognitive therapists and short-term workers, and a few psychoanalysts believe that the patient need only subject himself to the prescribed procedure and the results will follow more or less directly. Sometimes this does appear to happen. Many hysterical patients who are subjected to the classical psychoanalytical procedure unfold the neurosis and, to a large extent, its treatment. Some symptoms appear as vulnerable. But neither of those situations is the subject of these chapters, which are about finding and developing the other. In this process, the authority of therapists is a subject of exquisite difficulty.

The difficulty is a result of conflicting needs. On the one hand, the authority of the therapist can easily substitute for the freedom of the patient. The patient in search of himself, especially one profoundly out of touch, can easily replace himself with the therapist. Then the imputation and acceptance of power literally become self-defeating. On the other hand, psychotherapy can rarely afford to relinquish the authority of the therapist altogether. For example, demoralized people, which probably includes most who are searching for themselves, need to be in the presence of authority. This is what gives the work its start. Furthermore, the exploration and testing of the wishes a patient has for himself requires that he believe in the therapist's ability to accept or contain the often futile wanderings. One would wish to emulate Lincoln, who was described as having the hardness of steel and the softness of a cloud. Unfortunately, few of us meet those standards, and we need to find means to sustain both modesty and authority.[3]

Throughout I have suggested that the psychotherapist has to contain radically conflicting attitudes. This is technically necessary, and it also serves as an example to the patient, whose need for integration will pose the same demand. The willingness to be wrong is a rudimentary example of the same phenomenon, because one's readiness in this also implies the possibility of being right. These concurrent willingnesses are expressed by the idea of the hypothetical.

I want to approach the hypothetical accurately, but without too clean a sense of its meaning. To that end the following sentences of Lytton Strachey on Thomas Hardy's style seem useful.

> And he speaks, he does not sing. Or rather he talks—in the quiet voice of a modern man or woman, who finds it difficult as modern men and women do, to put into words exactly what is in his mind. He is incorrect; but then how unreal and artificial a thing is correctness! He fumbles, but it is that very fumbling that brings him so near ourselves.[4]

"It is that very fumbling that brings him so near ourselves." Hardy did not pretend to be absolutely correct. He suspected the personal and psychological matters at issue could only be approximated at best. He may even have intuited what is made explicit in modern physics—that precision and reliability are sometimes opposed because the very process of approaching and measuring introduces distortions of its own.

The hypothetical subsumes both these elements. It is an approach to truth, but not one opposed to the readiness, even eagerness, to be wrong, what is meant by the tentative and the provisional. The idea is not altogether clean because the respective amounts of truth and falsity can vary greatly, ranging from formal hypotheses to mere guesses or hunches. Projective statements entail the full scope of these extremes.

It is the power of the hypothetical to explore which lies at the heart of its role in science. It is an imaginative movement that invites a testing. Psychotherapy cannot afford to be without the hypothetical, since the material the patient produces spontaneously has many possible meanings that can be investigated only through hypotheses. This is the reason projective statements are a necessary addition to associative method. Many of the disputes and divisions of the psychoanalytic schools spring from the fundamental limits of using free association alone. The hypothetical function of projective statements allows therapists to pick their way among the sectarian biases. Moreover, in psychological work there is no sense in pretending to be correct or final, because we seldom are.

A British prime minister is reputed to have had a useful stammer. At the climax of a speech he would be unable to complete the final word he wanted, managing only its first or second syllable. The entire House of Commons, caught in the momentum of the prime minister's point, would join him in a mighty chorus to conclude the thought. In Strachey's words, he had brought them near himelf.

Setting an Example

There is another power in the willingness to be wrong which is a third source of the evocativeness of projective statements. Many patients need to be given permission to express what they feel, and consent is most powerfully implied by setting an example. It will be shown later how setting an example can also be *counter*-projective, since it removes from the therapist any projection of disapproval of expressiveness that his silence or authority may have drawn from the patient. Even in the absence of such inhibiting projections, the patient may need to be encouraged, given language, and shown the way.

There is an old recommendation about helping children overcome fears: not to push or urge the child, but to go forward yourself and pat or hold the feared object. Sometimes this also reveals that the child is reacting to the adult's fear and not his own. Note in the following exchange how my patient stays a step behind me in expressiveness, until he leaps ahead at the end.

H: You had to wonder if anybody knew.
P: No, everyone said she was perfect.
H: Perhaps you thought "I must be crazy?"
P: I always thought I was strange.
H: She was frightening.
P: I remember thinking, "Maybe I should lock the door."
H: Wouldn't she come in anyway?
P: She didn't knock. She made my sister unlock her door.
H: There was no stopping her.
P: I thought she must have a reason.
H: It would be easy to dislike her.
P: I forgot to kiss her one morning. She said, "Don't you love your mother?" I don't know what I felt.
H: Those black eyes.

P: Whenever my father and mother went out I'd think, "Maybe they'll be killed and never come back. I'll be free!"

Again, to ask or talk about his feelings would be to encourage their continued restraint in the form of intellectualizations. To set an example was to express "You can follow!"

Often love is even more difficult to express than hate, particularly when indicating to the therapist that the emotion is felt toward him. The patient may test the therapeutic bond, suicidal gestures being one example, in an attempt to discover if the therapist really cares in return. Sometimes it is enough to say, "You *love* me and naturally want me to love you," for the fact and frustration of that emotion to be expressed and its testing to stop. The point is, the patient may not dare voice it first or even admit it to himself. What undermines the familiar method of interpreting the patient's resistances is that even when they have been accurately interpreted, the fear of disappointment may not abate, in part because the patient is not clearly experiencing the therapist's attitude toward love; he may be even more fearful of rejection because the therapist talks around it. Also, the patient is often right.

This is apparent when the therapist resists speaking directly of love because he is embarrassed by the patient's feelings for him and doesn't know how to respond. The patient *is* in danger of having his love rejected. Here the magnificent idea of transference love can be pressed into the service of the therapist's resistance. "You do not love me but, instead, the memory of your mother" is often at once true and hurtful. To say joyfully and thankfully, "You love me," can admit love onto the plane of the relationship and do so without criticism. The transferential elements will follow.

In addition, a fresh use of projective statements can be reached. The hypothetical may be limit-setting. The patient says or implies, "If you are accepting of love, why don't you love me back, dine with me, sleep with me?" If the analyst is to be therapist and not lover or spouse, his projective mark is plain as paint and as needful of color in the saying. "Would that I could! Would that the work made room for them both!"

Of course, this very "showing the way" must elicit some reservations. Are we not putting ideas into the minds of patients? Are we indicating to them what we want, as opposed to what they want? Are we showing a basic lack of respect for patients by abrogating their leadership and presuming their views? Nothing stands out more sharply in the whole history of psychoanalysis than respect for patients, the real waiting on them that the almost unlimited, silent attention of analysis reflects. Once therapists are liberated to talk, it is also unlikely that they will keep the same balance of interest in what the patients say. Many therapists, enthralled by their own cleverness, will be much more interested in their own remarks than in the patients'. Nor can we hope for a great deal from the admonition to talk only when the patient will not, because such a maxim says nothing about how long to wait. There is only one honest answer to the objection, and it will not change every mind. It applies equally to psychotherapeutic and medical practices: every new technique carries drawbacks and creates complications. The additions can only be evaluated in terms of their specific indications and overall effects. Once the doctor learns that he can draw blood and gain priceless information from it, he has that much less time to examine, and a proportionately stronger temptation to take more.

The Democratization of Therapy

To the strength of detail, of the hypothetical, and of setting an example can be added the democratizing power of projective statements. As already suggested, they are equalizing. It is helpful to make some statements offhandedly, almost to oneself, so that shy or suspicious people do not feel pressured. The most tactful question in the world is still inquisitive and requests an answer. To some measure, it carries the memories of all questions that could not be answered or were shaming or damning to acknowledge. Sensitive clinicians have always known this. Recall the rising inflection at the end of a statement, as in "n'est-ce pas?" mentioned earlier. Statements then become only half-questions, saying, "You can answer or correct me if you like, but I'm not pressing you." It avoids sounding like a district attorney.[5] These further particulars are not trivial. I quoted Napoleon on the power of details, which led to a connection between battles and psychotherapy. Therapists also marshal powerful forces and then find that these can be turned, often suddenly, against them.

Nothing turns these forces more decisively than the imbalance in most psychotherapeutic and psychoanalytic work. When the therapist questions, he puts himself in the position of judging the patient. Can the patient answer, above all, correctly or non-pathologically? If the therapist waits, he perforce stands in judgment; the material is brought to him as to an investigator or judge, even to one who may decide whether he will receive or accept at all.

Therapists who deny this should recall their own experiences of treatment or consultations with other analysts and supervisors. Such experiences are unbalanced because, inevitably, correctness, goodness, and even healthiness adhere to the therapist or supervisor, while at least the possibility of the opposite attributes are connected with the patient or student. As a rule, such an inequality is enormously provocative of transference, especially of negative reactions transferred from the innumerable experiences everyone shares as child and student. One of the great difficulties of psychopathological judgment is deciding how much these transferences are evoked by the clinical situation or how much they are created.

Projective statements have the merit of putting the therapist's fallibility forward first—so it is the patient who judges and corrects. Moreover, the therapist sets an example of happy receptivity; he is delighted to be corrected and have the record set straight. The truth is served. Later we will see the opportunities that projective statements provide for a fresh approach to countertransference. Suffice it here to celebrate the democratization of psychotherapeutic work they encourage, which leads to a real possibility of exchange.

Freud surmised from his study of dreams that the deepest levels of mental life operated under an ancient, primitive canon of justice called the talion principle: "An eye for an eye, a tooth for a tooth." If this is so, the usual imbalance of clinical work is poorly suited to engaging these submerged forms of thought. Perhaps even what has been met and called resistance is to some measure only this talion principle mobilized into the therapeutic situation. The deepest levels of mind may say, "If you refuse to give to me, then I will not give to you."

Projective statements are free offerings meant to be taken, amended, or set aside. By their readiness of offering, they invite a reciprocal attitude of generosity and freedom. Use of such statements will sometimes turn resistance into cooperation and alliance. The evocative powers of projective statements are directed both at finding the other and, by means of the hypothetical element, testing what has been discovered. The closely related counterassumptive language we look at next provides a way to control an invasive other.

Counterassumptive Statements

Counterassumptive statements are comments made by therapists that unsettle assumptions they feel being made about them by their patients—suppositions, say, of the therapists' omniscience. It is seldom wise to confront these assumptions directly because patients are usually unaware of them and might regard such a charge as an accusation of madness. Counterassumptive statements shake assumptions without making them a matter for debate.

The earliest instances of shaking assumptions I encountered were the result of comic or arch behavior. One therapist discovered himself in the presence of gross overestimations of his ability, which harbored all the danger of fostering great expectations that could only lead to ultimate disappointment. So he made it a point to forget the patient's name, stumble clumsily while showing the patient out, and even fall off his chair. Another therapist declared early on, "I hope I don't make a bigger mess of things than your last doctor." Both therapists intended to reduce their patients' expectations to reasonable levels. The primary difficulty with these tactics is that most workers find them too bizarre to imagine acting out. A more systematic and less idiosyncratic language is needed.

111

Signaling Attitudes

I suspect that some women learn earlier and more thoroughly than men how to signal attitudes and to exercise subtle controls. This is because women are often the recipients of social actions denying them the power that makes direct confrontation permissible. Consider the plight of women caught in ostensibly romantic situations with unattractive men. It may not be prudent simply to say "Goodnight" at the end of the evening. Everyone knows men who pride themselves not only on their physical superiority but on never taking no for an answer. It is better to signal early and repeatedly that little will be forthcoming, that the man will be fortunate to leave with an unbruised ego. The evening had best begin coolly so that it can end that way.

Unfortunately, much of the social training women receive moves them in the opposite direction, toward enthusiasm, compliance, and dependence. These in turn condition the aggressive man to expect his way. One result is that frank women, who simply say goodnight, are damned when they should be praised, and dependent women, who have not learned to exercise indirect controls, are put in humiliating, dangerous situations.

I once worked for a man who had extraordinary skill in controlling people's expectations. A subordinate would enter his office intent on expressing a protest or eliciting a favor, only to leave without having accomplished either, but no longer angry or hopeful. Often the person forgot what he came for. Two skills had been exercised. The wishes of the subordinate had been sensed immediately; it was unnecessary to tell this man what you wanted. He then assumed an attitude that was at once understanding and very firm, which literally turned off the subordinate's planned behavior. The subordinate wanted to be promoted; he encountered a polite and slightly pitying attitude, implying he would be lucky to keep his job. Or the subordinate entered the office furious —the boss would be made to pay! Five minutes later, he emerged smiling and deferential or even laughing and enthusiastic. His mood had been sensed the moment he crossed the threshold. He was either greeted by a larger thundercloud than he carried himself or found his rage deflected and discharged. Proteus had changed his shape, and few subordinates were able to cling.

In *Call for the Dead* John Le Carré has his hero Smiley handle an intrusive and unpleasant interviewer by imagining that the man has thick fur on his face. So as not to be intimidated he balances the great power of the interviewer with an imaginative correction. He creates a free space around himself in which he can exercise his individuality. We might say Smiley made the interviewer human, if it were not that he turned him into an animal. The issue was self-preservation; the tools were perception, imagination, and attitude.

Shaking Assumptions

Everyday speech includes a device that is powerfully and simply counterassumptive without being contrived or clever. It is the attribution of a quality in the guise of a warning proverb or maxim. In the presence of great expectations an example would be, "Hope springs eternal," said rather mordantly, which implies to the patient, "You have the wonderful quality of hopefulness, but beware." Proverbs address common dangers, for instance the risk of certain disappointment from entertaining unrealistic hopes, and are psychotherapeutically helpful because their common usage depersonalizes them; the therapist is merely borrowing from the universal stock of wisdom.

Another example deals with the opposite situation. In my experience, therapists suffer much less than they might because of patients' low expectations, since such patients are grateful for any positive results. But a therapist is sometimes assumed to be stupid or predictably useless, an attitude that can be wearing. A Persian proverb states, "Contempt is able to penetrate even the shell of the tortoise." As a rule, contemptuous people are unaware of their contempt and find it unattractive in others, so again the assumption must be handled indirectly.

The observer may wish to say, "Pride goes before a fall," but the reasons for refraining are instructive. Note in the first example that the patient is not accused of idealization or overhopefulness, only of that solid virtue, hopefulness. Yet the second accusation, of pride, borders on a return charge of contempt. Furthermore, the warning is direct, indeed baleful; hope was only said to "spring eternal." Thus the proverb concerning pride fails on both counts: it is overly accusing and it is too directly admonitory. It does not shake, but confronts.

In different words, "Hope springs eternal" gently expresses what the therapist perceives in the patient's attitude. On the other hand, "Pride goes before a fall" declares the opinion of the therapist, which may be the direct opposite of the patient's and is therefore antipathetic.

As discussed in relation to simple empathic statements, contempt is a difficult attitude to share, expecially when it is directed at you. The empathic task becomes easier if the contempt is aimed at outsiders. This last can be utilized psychotherapeutically once the therapist acknowledges and puts outside himself a characteristic of himself or his profession that sane people would regard with skepticism. Skepticism, in turn, has many uses and is as readily preferred to contempt as hopefulness is to overestimation. Now we are on our way. The possibility of empathy with skepticism is in place. The therapist should be able to identify something about his professional work which evokes skepticism. It only remains to pick up these two points and give them a slight proverbial shaking.

Not so long ago doctors were regarded as almost more dangerous than the diseases they were supposed to treat. As a result we have many once-familiar sayings that express skepticism toward the medical profession. Perhaps the most damning is a German proverb, "A young doctor means a new graveyard," which today could be more appropriately phrased, "A young doctor means a rise in the cost of living." More serviceable is Ben Franklin's "God heals and the doctor takes the fee." This supports the skepticism of the patient, acknowledges the therapist's limitations, and at the same time undermines the patient's contempt. One might protest that it supports the contempt. In fact it does not because, for a moment, the patient's attitude is expressed, even a little caricatured, so that it is not so solidly in place; it has been seen.

An often subtle but pervasive attitude many patients bring to therapy can be termed the search for personal error or evil. The patient is looking to find something bad about himself. This may be a subtle attitude partly because it is difficult to separate from the intelligent search for neurotic trends and conflicts. Naturally, the patient's reception of the therapist's discoveries and interpretations will be colored by this attitude. What the therapist takes to be some patients' receptivity and insightfulness may be nothing more than their satisfaction in having found something actually wrong. Sometimes this attitude is blatant; then we recognize depressive self-depreciation and self-punitiveness. But there are many less extreme, often mildly depressive characters who are just selling themselves short. They think of themselves as jerks or slobs, waiting to be everywhere unmasked. The therapist is expected to see and agree with the judgment, however much the agreement is resented. Later, I shall take up a full-blown psychotherapeutic attack on such attitudes, with their apparatus of identification with hostile internalized figures and the ready projection of the hostile figures outward. Suffice it here to suggest how one shakes these attitudes a little, begins to bring them into perspective, and avoids letting them settle too complacently on the relationship.

The basic form of the disconfirming response is: "Yes, I know, you're a real dope," stated skeptically. The patient's image has been received and verbalized, with the skepticism of the therapist indicated. Yet a proverbial rendering demonstrates why this basic form is generally unusable, at the same time exposing the various counterassumptive elements.

In my first example, the idealizing patient puts a burden of hopefulness on the therapist. In the second, the contemptuous patient does the opposite. The third example asks the therapist, in turn, to be contemptuous. In each case the therapist needs to translate the patient's expectations into an acceptable form, and then throw a dash of salt on those expectations. "Yes, I know, you're a real dope" *is* usable, but only after a firm relationship has been established. The expectations of the patient are crudely expressed, and the therapist is likely to be experienced as confirming the patient's expectations by ridiculing him, certainly no dash of salt.

An acceptable form of meeting the patient's expectation of contempt can be called modesty. Tell someone who is busy berating himself that he seems "modest" and the person often feels a little reconciled to himself. There are interesting reasons why this reconciliation is not always forthcoming. Lord Chesterfield advised his son, "Modesty is the only sure bait when you angle for praise." He could just as sensibly have warned his son of the opposite reaction. William Hazlitt wrote, a generation after Chesterfield, "A modest man is the natural butt of impertinence." Chesterfield no doubt did not mean by modesty what Hazlitt did—true modesty. Chesterfield's letters are largely advice on strategies, lessons in simulation; modesty as a pose elicits very different responses than modesty as a quality. I make this point because clinical self-depreciation consists of varying mixtures of manipulation and genuine expressiveness; the two are not exclusive. Yet which is the counterassumptive to address—the expectation of receiving praise for not being vain or the expectation of being thought deficient or evil? Note how in everyday life the decision is made automatically, through the contagion of affects. The truly modest person conveys the feeling of being deficient and thereby becomes the "butt of impertinence." In contrast, the manipulative person elicits the very feeling of confidence he has been able to put into his strategem. The ideal would be to address both assumptions, but that requires finding a common denominator of manipulativeness and expressiveness, which seem so opposed on the surface. Of course we do not have to address both at once; we may sense, again through our own emotional responses to the patient, the relative amounts of each present and then address the predominant feeling. Nevertheless, the search for an encompassing formula illustrates the range and power of counterassumptive statements.

The expectations of praise and condemnation do have in common the desire for a response. If the contents of these appeals have opposite signs, they also share a turning over of power and judgment to the therapist. In this respect the manipulator and the depressed person come together. How can one express this turning over to the other in a way that is not denigrating, that is, indeed, admiring? The fact that people need one another is something neither to be despised nor to be admired; it is simply a fact of life. The acknowledgment of that need is surely admirable, but does the admiration extend to the need to be praised and blamed? In one sense, yes. We need to see ourselves through other eyes, even if what we would like to see bears little relationship to what is seen.

The counterassumptive statement will hospitably recognize the desire to be judged and then lightly undercut the expectation of the judgment's safety. The person expecting praise should feel a little unsure, and the person expecting to seem foolish should feel mildly praised. I cannot think of an appropriate maxim, but let me construct one. Imagine two travelers, a rich man and a poor man, arriving late on a stormy night at an isolated cottage. One expects to be greeted warmly, fed, and bedded down; the other believes he will be thrown to the rain and wind. The cottage owner is neither rich enough to feed two strangers nor mean enough to turn them away. Yet he does a certain miraculous justice by them both, and, like most miracles, it is a miracle principally in the speaking. He tells the travelers to come in out of the foul weather, explaining that he has no extra food but they are welcome to take shelter for the night. Handing them two empty sacks to use as bedding, he utters our new proverb. It is a gift and a warning to all those who look to others either for everything or nothing: "The man who asks puts himself at another's mercy; the man who gives disappoints the rich and does not prepare the poor man for tomorrow."

Even the most desperate clinician, even the worker still comfortable asking the patient to do serial sevens and to consider living in glass houses, as the psychological examination dictates, will hesitate at this stark extremity. But he may see the point. You want to shake the patient's expectations a little, to cool the rich man's avarice and to comfort the poor man while preparing him for the "impertinence" he will continue to receive.

Moving the Observer

David, a handsome lawyer, well-dressed and a little grave, treated me from the start with great deference and respect. Because he had a besieged, almost haunted look to him, I believed, instead, that he was afraid. I would not have been surprised if he thought I was some kind of dangerous lunatic who had to be handled with care. It soon appeared that he was also bewildered. He would begin his legal cases with dispatch, organize his thoughts carefully, contact appropriate people and make suggestions, only to find, often suddenly, that the case had been terminated, been given to someone else, or made him the subject of angry attack. This had happened repeatedly. He came for help when his wife and the chief partner of his firm furiously insisted, and he didn't know why.

This man's deliberate, almost stately manner might have seemed pompous and affected to many people. He was not sensitive or shrewd in judging others, and I suspected that he was seen as invasive or overpowering. Yet it was not obvious why the feelings he provoked should be so harsh or the rejections so decisive. David said that for many years he had attempted to placate his wife and that he saw himself as kindly and helpful. At the same time, he bitterly resented her. Deference can provoke rage if it is followed by pomposity or invasiveness. Was it the combination of fearfulness and "lord of the manor" stateliness that made him so provocative?

Later work with this patient would expose early experiences and personal tendencies that made understandable both the fear and the pomposity. But the subsequent work could not have been possible until I forestalled in treatment the very reactions that were threatening to destroy his whole life. It was also likely that any reinforcement of his fear or pomposity would undo the value of historical insight. David's assumption of my dangerousness would be reinforced by offensive or eccentric behavior on my part. Yet, if I were quiet and polite, he might regard me safely as his servant. The counterassumptive attitudes and statements would have to offset both danger and safety.

I could not expect David to acknowledge either side. He gave no sign of being aware of his feelings or manner. He did not know that he did not know—he never complained of being bewildered. I thought he felt wounded and depreciated, all the while maintaining a stance of proud composure. He had been referred by a law teacher who had once been his ideal. I thought he came to me as he may have approached the teacher, hoping once again to be respected and understood. He came regularly from a distant city, to avoid any possibility that his seeking help would be known and not respected.

David's apparent search for the protection and values of an idealized figure could explain his deference and fear. Would I, in fact, respect him, or would he be subjected to a fresh attack? It could also account for some of his stateliness, to give me a reason to respect him. Again, I was running a risk if I either failed his hopes or realized his dreams: I could disappoint and lose him or enmesh him in a new adoration. Furthermore, his possible search for an ideal was flattering, coming from one self-important professional man to another. It would have been delightful for me to assume that I was both "exactly what the doctor ordered" and the doctor who did the ordering. Bewildered people are the natural prey of cult leaders, whether religious or psychotherapeutic, teachers who claim to know what others should be and do. This impressive man was a good catch. The difficulty was that, much as he might want to idealize me, I might not be what the doctor ordered; he had to find that for himself. Later I found out about the particular person in his adolescence who had given him the stately ideal. That person had been seized upon, to his apparent delight. No doubt that had also offset David's fear and bewilderment. Still it was not a free, open choice. This was what I wanted to give him.

The tasks of restoring David's morale while not dictating his ideals paralleled the counterassumptive tasks of not increasing his fear and, at the same time, avoiding reinforcement of his pomposity. The first psychotherapeutic task, therefore, was a "holding open," or keeping away, not allowing him to find something in me he could readily idolize and imitate. Perhaps part of his fear was based on just this prospect of surrendering to me. It would not be safe for the patient to see more of me until he began to wonder who and where he was, rather than reaching blindly out. Then the shoe would be on the other foot: I would be the one to worry about my assumptions as to his value or offensiveness.

At the same time, this bewildered man could not enjoy or even continue the therapeutic work if his bewilderment were to increase. He had to be offered something in exchange for the prolonging of his confusion. Moreover, this "something" would have to sail the narrow channel between a fresh imposition of ideals and the thousand empty gestures of help that bewildered people so often receive. For example, it would not be safe to offer the lawyer a "legal solution," that he had somehow broken the rules of his institution or marriage and therefore invited wrath. It would not be wise to offer this even if it were deserved, precisely because it would impose a notion he himself should come up with. Suppose he had broken the rules; it was still his decision that these were the rules and institutions for him. The point is, he could not be offered any solution at all; he was going to have to create it. For a long time we moved about among the possibilities. The best of these were not distant islands to be sailed toward, but more like anchors already on board that one pitched out to see if they held.

I stated earlier that therapists need to throw a dash of salt on the patient's expectations. In moving the observer, there is the same searching for what is acceptable to the patient and the same possibility of shaking what is found. The quest takes on an element of drama when it is part of the patient's search for himself, a search that the therapist wants to prolong in order to find the person. For example, how did I know that this patient was really bewildered? Perhaps he feigned an ignorance of the causes of his difficulties. He may have feared that anything he knew and reported about his mistakes would provoke my ridicule. I have already suggested that he seemed afraid of me; bewilderment could have been his protection, like the black ink of the octopus. If this were true, then he should appear less confused as he felt less afraid. Change my fearsome shape, the hypothesis went, and look for what remained of his confusion. I might also watch those fearful eyes.

But it was difficult to ascertain what it was about me that frightened David. One of James Thurber's cartoons shows a patient sitting up on the couch and pointing a gun at the analyst. The caption reads, "Doctor, you know too much." Was the lawyer afraid that I knew too much, or did he confuse me with the irascible, unpredictable mother he gradually described? Maybe I truly was fearsome—after all, I did sometimes feel like deflating him. On the other hand, he may simply have been demonstrating the usual uneasiness people feel when meeting strangers, particularly psychiatric strangers.[1] I was the one who should have been confused.

In fact, I felt confident and clear. I was in my own office, doing what I had done a hundred times before; moreover, I felt challenged by this man, and somehow equal to the challenge. Yet my clarity is not so comprehensible. What was I clear about? This seems at least as mysterious as David's apparent bewilderment and fear. What I felt clear about was my uncertainty. Further, I was sure that the uncertainty could be gradually lessened, although it would never disappear. Certainty is not in the nature of scientific work, nor is it a term one associates with art. In seeing a number of murky problems before us, though, progress had already been made.

Psychotherapist and patient can be compared to strangers boarding an unfamiliar vehicle. Either or both may drive; either or both may choose the destination. Some therapists drive taxis, ready to go anywhere the patient asks, provided the driver knows how to get there. Others are like bus drivers, with a fixed route. Still others, myself included, try to share both the driving and the choice of destination. Such a sharing is exciting, partly because of the high level of uncertainty throughout. Anyone who has been in a taxi or bus that gets lost knows the rapidity with which distinctions between passenger and driver disappear.

At the outset the lawyer and I were not lost; getting lost would happen many times, but later. This gave me my first counterassumptive opportunity. I said, less a question than as a rhetorical statement of uncertainty, "Where to go?" The emphasis was on "where," with more than a hint of resignation in the "to go." He immediately seemed less fearful. I had used a rhetorical question that was at the same time an imitative statement—his bewilderment was shared. I also had countered the possible assumption that I would control his life—he was a participant in this. Further, I had not criticized him—he was not told that he had made a fine mess of things. Finally, I had avoided the reinforcement of David's stateliness. I was not being pompous myself or offering to go where he suggested. We were to mull things over together.

Throughout our journey, this proud man would look to me for the choice of destination. Sometimes he would do so openly, in a graceful gesture of self-deferral. More often he was furtive, fearing guidance as much as he wanted it. This modesty I often acknowledged, at the same time casting doubt on the value of modesty when choosing life goals. Even more important was to shake any view of me that seemed to be solidifying: I had to change shape.

Modesty was wonderfully appealing to David in the wake of his professional and marital defeats. It seemed a sensible, attractive posture for a man who had been widely accused of error and pride. It avoided pitting him against me at a time when he was eager to defer. It also seemed "patiently" deportment; he, the fellow professional, could come down off his high horse.

I played it back and forth. When nothing subtle could seem to dislodge his too modest assumptions, I quoted some words of May Sarton's: "If one does not have wild dreams of achievement, there is no spur even to get the dishes washed."[2] If he seemed full of the old days, when nothing was beyond him, I recalled how little any of us achieves our brightest hopes. At one point he thought he had found me out in my career at Harvard. He said, "You must know how to build an empire among the sharks and whales." I didn't want to tell him that the only empire I had built was in my head, since that might also become his empire. Neither could he be left with his original assumption. Here again was a narrow channel to navigate. My response was, "Well, I hope you could survive longer among the sharks and whales than I could." The implications were clear: good luck, it was not for me. I offered no encouragement either, since I was far from confident about his ability to survive. David was not supposed to find me; he was supposed to find himself. The hope was that if he clung long enough, the answers would come—as they did.

It was she who first gave me the idea that a person does not (as I had imagined) stand motionless and clear before our eyes with his merits, his defects, his plans, his intentions with regard to us exposed on his surface, like a garden at which, with all its borders spread out before us, we gaze through a railing; but is a shadow which we can never succeed in penetrating.

MARCEL PROUST

Counterprojective Statements

Psychotherapy is mutually subversive: therapist and patient project on one another. This does not mean only misperceiving and misunderstanding, but a real changing or subverting of the other. The empathic task of finding and assuming the viewpoint of the patient reduces this tendency on the side of the therapist. What can be done about subversion of the therapist by the patient? We cannot expect an equal empathic effort from the patient.

Projection follows attention, and projective statements, as a rule, direct attention away from the clinical relationship. So any projective statement would tend to reduce projections on the therapist. Connected here too is the phenomenon of strangers who become easily friendly while watching a fire or a parade.

This counterprojective power of projective statements can be increased by two measures: speaking about whatever is being projected on the therapist, and doing so with some of the feeling that the patient has toward the projection. Essentially, the therapist positions himself beside the patient and shares the feelings and attitudes toward the projection.

An illustration is the everyday reaction to someone responding to an acute insult or pain—for example, stubbing an injured toe. Stubbing your toe typically results in anger toward the object, blaming it, even wanting to kick the offending object again; this is the normal response. An observer standing close to the offending object may also be resented, a stimulus generalization or transference phenomenon. Moreover, the hurt person often resents questioning, and sometimes implies that he thinks the observer must know what is wrong, which suggests a temporary loss of ego boundaries. The treatment of such small, paranoid psychoses is, first, empathy with the pain and then alliance against the object. A friend can be quickly made by kicking the offending object for the injured person. Professionals are probably better off talking. Just as certain exclamations, "How painful!" or "That must have hurt," are the prototypic form of empathic speech, so another exclamation, "That damn chair," is the prototype of counterprojective speech.

In short, counterprojective statements move attention, along with critical figures or objects, and share hostile and other feelings. We shall also note that it is a way of seeing by means of the shadows, by means of figures thrown on the screen in front of both therapist and patient.

Counterprojective Devices

I emphasize language, but there are many devices commonly used in psychotherapy that have the same effect. Perhaps the best known is the use of play objects in child analysis. The child's projections, so often of a global and delusional extent, are thereby deflected onto the play objects, allowing the therapist to be more realistically seen. Winnicott developed another technique for children that invites a still closer comparison with what is being described.[1] In his squiggle game, one person makes lines or marks on a piece of paper, and the other is invited to add additional lines or marks, perhaps to complete specific representations. Indeed, Winnicott's technique might also be named what I have termed the "making of marks and remarks," or projective speech.

In Aaron Beck's cognitive therapy, an image is elicited that accompanies a symptom, say an image of large, dangerous people associated with anxiety.[2] This is then put out before the therapist and patient, to establish its pervasiveness, its difference from reality, and later its experiential roots. The emphasis is first on fantasy, as with projective testing, and then on experience and differences from contemporary reality. We can ask what determines whether the resulting material is fact or fantasy. While learning to administer psychological tests, I noticed that both the Rorschach and Thematic Apperception Test cards produced fantasies, but the latter produced factual material as well. Was this because the TAT cards were more realistic? I think it is generally true that the more actual the stimulus, the more factual the resulting material will be. David Garfield has called this an example of birds of a feather flocking together.[3]

Note that the selection of fantasy or reality is also a sectarian matter, particularly between psychoanalytic and social psychiatrists. In analytic training, one used to be told that only the patient's ideas about reality mattered. I suspect that for many therapists the relation between fantasy and reality was established at a time when reality seemed stable and fantasy was fantastic. Now the relation between fantasy and reality is often reversed, fantasy seeming a pale version of reality.

Many students of group therapy and psychodrama have also used externalizing or distancing devices. Fritz Perls emphasized them.[4] For example, he recommended designating a chair in the room as containing the patient's mother; therapist and patient could then address her together. This element of his therapeutic work seems to overshadow even the empathic and cathartic ones so prominent in his suggestions. As in Beck's method, transference management takes a lesser, even inadvertent role.

Murray Bowen's family therapy is also prominently counterprojective. For instance: "The new effort was to work out problems in the already existing intense relationships within the family and to specifically avoid actions and techniques that facilitate and encourage the therapeutic relationship with the therapist."[5] The therapist should be neutral in order to prevent the development of transference entanglements, which were to be worked out between family members themselves. Somewhat similar to play therapy, transference is to be resolved "out there." Bowen continues:

> My best operating emotional distance from the family, even when sitting physically close, is the point I can "see" the emotional process flowing back and forth between them. The human phenomenon is usually as humorous and comical as it is serious and tragic. The right distance is the point it is possible to see either the serious or the humorous side . . . It is necessary for the therapist to keep his focus on the process between the two. If he finds himself focusing on the content of what is being said, it is evident that he has lost sight of the process and he is emotionally entangled on the content issue.

What he calls the "magic of family therapy" is the process of "externalizing the thinking of each spouse": each is to examine the other's transference, feelings are avoided, and the emphasis is on facts and ideas. It is possible that Bowen's capacity to elicit this material depends on his having moved projections away from himself.

Much of the therapeutic action of "paradoxical intention" can also be termed counterprojective. The therapist typically places himself on the side of the forbidden wish. If the patient is obsessed with the idea of throwing a brick through a plate-glass window, he is encouraged to do so. The forbidden wish is empathically expressed, and prohibiting forces that may be projected onto the therapist are counterprojected. In short, the patient's internal conflict is not supported.

As a final example, Otto Kernberg includes what he calls "deflection" among his recommendations for the treatment of borderline patients:

> The main characteristics of this proposed modification in the psychoanalytic procedure are . . . systematic elaboration of the manifest and latent negative transference without attempting to achieve full genetic reconstructions on the basis of it, followed by "deflection" of the manifest negative transference away from the therapeutic interaction through systematic examination of it in the patient's relations with others.[6]

We could also speak of supporting certain defenses, such as displacement and externalization. However, from the viewpoint of social psychiatry, the issue of what is defensive on the one hand or accurately attributive on the other depends upon the separation of fact from fantasy.

These ideas are as old as the hills. Wise clinicians have always known that there are many people in the room; the wisest have formed some way of saying to obstreperous patients, "Your mother must be in the room." Shrewd parents do the same thing: they will spell out their difficult day so that the children will not expect too much on a tired evening.

Uniting Medium and Message

Working away from the patient may be necessary if the patient is invasive, or when closeness would encourage too great an intimacy or grandiose hopes. The medium should support the message. Because the actual language that therapists use in their work has been so largely neglected, the medium in which therapeutic messages are carried too often contradicts the messages themselves. This is painfully evident when, for example, the bidding of "be spontaneous" contradicts the very freedom prescribed.[7] This is only the tip of the iceberg, however. More commonly, clear explanations and incisive comments about a patient's excessive dependence or hopefulness inadvertently reinforce the qualities they are intended to reduce. What we do speaks louder than what we say—with such a helpful and knowing therapist, why not hope, and depend?[8]

Patients may often wonder, "Why doesn't my therapist do more when he is trained, paid for, and knows my suffering? Why is so much left to me?" In the case of the patient about to be considered, the contradiction was unexpressed because of his expectation that the therapist would someday do something; the patient had only to wait. In the meantime, this belief led the patient to do very little. Implicit in these attitudes were two projections: the therapist had a secret knowledge or power he could impart, and he had some undetermined reason for withholding it.

Note that such projections could not be dealt with directly. Largely unrecognized by the patient, if interpreted they would probably have been denied. Suppose the interpretations did by chance reach the patient: they would surely confirm his magical expectations of the "clever therapist" or, if taken on faith, his own dependency. Working away from the patient can reduce these contradictions of medium and message, as we shall see. In addition, the material will demonstrate how the declarative mode can move attention away from the clinical relationship and with it, specific projections.

In making the following interventions, I decided not to let the transference develop freely to the discovery of the paternal magic and its withholding for mother, which were later reached. I believed that the patient's projections would be disruptive if left unchecked, possibly resulting in a paranoid transference psychosis. I also decided against an empathic elaboration of the patient's helplessness and hopelessness, although this too was partly achieved later.

Bart: Why don't you clarify this? You know me very well, I'm confused. [The intuitive association was, "The patient wants to see my penis," because one of the patient's major symptoms was a preoccupation with "other men" and their penises, in his triangular relationships. I didn't say this, though, because if it "took" it would again seem like magic to the patient and reinforce little-boy expectations. If it did not, it would only add to the confusion he complained of.]

Havens: That's right. [I am attempting to put the patient's confusion "out there," by saying in effect, "Let's get this clear; it is confusing." There is also some acknowledgment of the confusion and irritation.]

B: I can't do it alone. [The patient might have been returned to the past, into his alternately indulged and besieged childhood, with an empathic "Often you were alone." But I wanted to deal first with the gradually surfacing indignation at my withholding, which was too real to be handled as only transference. Nor would it have been wise to invite a therapeutic collaboration of examining it: "Let's look at why you feel indignant now." The patient might have cooperated in this on the basis of the therapist's authority; but again his submissiveness and dependence would have been exploited.]

H: Neither your boss nor the girlfriend has clarified things either.

B: They haven't.

H: Everywhere you look, no one helps. [Said empathically.]

B: But you're supposed to.

H: I suppose your parents were too.

B: They didn't.

H: No wonder you want someone to take their place. [Both empathic and externalizing. The therapist shares the patient's understandable yearning and locates one source outside the treatment.]

First I try to preserve the patient's independence and self-respect; I don't want to reward the regressive entitlement to be "properly taken care of this time." Understandable as that demand is, its satisfaction would imply that the patient could not perform these functions himself and, more dangerously, that the therapist is under an obligation to compensate for what the parents had neglected. This could lead to an escalating series of demands.

My second intention is to move the angry feelings generated by boss, girlfriend, and parents away from myself and "out there," to be examined—a counterprojection. If successful, this will allow Bart to be more realistic about the treatment. He should also be able to see more clearly his expectations toward others. In fact, just after this exchange, he inquired of himself whether he did not ask too much of the treatment and was therefore disappointed. He also said that he remembered fantasizing that both boss and girlfriend would be far better than father and mother. I didn't support Bart's suspicion that he had expected too much of boss and girlfriend. I couldn't know whether this was indeed the case or, equally possible, if the patient had chosen individuals for boss and girlfriend who would disappoint him, as his parents had. In other words, I didn't know if the patient's difficulty was one of repetitive, perhaps neurotic expectations or a neurotic re-creation of an original family scene.[9] So I couldn't explain to Bart what the difficulty was. Indeed, he may have picked and stayed with a therapist who was also determined to withhold from him! Above all, I wanted to escape the vexing decision of whether I should give the patient more or less, which any attempt to work by means of a "corrective emotional experience" would have demanded. Nor could I work by providing interpetations, that is, explanations to the patient's rational ego. Beyond the issue of their correctness, they might be seen as gratifying gifts and, consequently, justify the demands of the patient. Moreover, they would have concentrated attention on me, with the danger of bringing more of the patient's projections back.

Hence avoiding double messages and moving patients' projections are sometimes identical processes. This is because the medium of the message may reinforce a projection that undercuts the message. In Bart's case, by supporting his expectations of my helpfulness, I would have weakened his need to help himself. Moving this projection away avoided a contradictory communication.

Attack on the Projection

Transference psychosis is a patient's distorted view of the therapist that reaches psychotic proportions. "Psychotic proportions" has no precise extent, no more than the distinction between neurosis and psychosis does. Yet each psychological function registers the idea of psychosis in a roughly discernible way. Cognition is affected to a delusional extent; the patient becomes convinced of the therapist's deviltry or greatness. This conviction is delusional precisely because it does not respond to fact or reason. Perception may even be affected in an hallucinatory fashion, where the therapist comes to resemble the father or mother. The effects on emotion are also dramatic; in psychotic reactions the hate or love is intense, overpowering. This usually has another result, the most dramatic of all. A patient in the grip of a positive transference psychosis is fully capable of appearing at the therapist's breakfast table and shouldering his wife aside.

As a rule, such states develop gradually. When intense hate or love toward the therapist is evident from the start, all these phenomena will be present—but the names are not the same. We speak of psychoses, not transference psychoses. What gives transference psychoses their scientific interest is the opportunity they offer to study and sometimes correct psychotic phenomena that occur in the therapist's office, and that develop slowly enough to permit a detailed understanding. Many believe that such developments indicate a preexistent psychosis, or at least a psychotic propensity, and deny their occurrence in the case of people seemingly neurotic. This is not my impression. Not only is it tautological to assume that everyone who has a psychotic reaction is inherently psychotic, it also overlooks a fact of great importance. The provocation that some therapeutic situations offer the patient has such a divisive and disorganizing potential that it might drive anyone mad.

This is not an isolated reference to the seductions and aggressions that infuse all aspects of life, including the treatment scene. I specifically cite the great excitement and promise so often aroused at the onset of treatment. If this condition is sharply reversed by a change in the therapist's situation, the patient's having to move elsewhere, or the therapist's sudden fear of too much closeness, it can result in disorganization and psychosis.

By definition, psychoses and transference psychoses both resist interpretative resolution. In fact, efforts at explaining to patients their distortion of the therapist regularly exacerbate the psychotic process. It is not difficult to understand why. People in the grip of strong feelings seldom appreciate having these feelings labeled as inappropriate or misplaced; they may rightly sense and resent the accusation of madness. What ensues is nothing other than an argument that, like many arguments, reinforces the resentments and misunderstandings of both parties. Vigorous interpretations can transform mild transference misunderstandings into dangerous transference psychoses, which may not be a troubling or surprising result to either party. The patient feels confirmed in his attitude toward the therapist, and the therapist will regard any suspicions he had about the severity of the patient's condition as accurate.

The empathic statement is "It's infuriating," not "You are mad." The counterprojective force of the empathic statement is increased by two steps: the object of the rage or love is mentioned, and the emotion is expressed with a vehemence to match the patient's. The statement "It's infuriating" becomes "So-and-so is infuriating," said with force. The ability of counterprojective speech to reduce rage and love to manageable proportions, and not to increase them, should be confirmed by skeptical readers from their own experience. There is only one cautionary note: be sure that the expression of emotions is empathic. If the expression is attributive and descriptive, the patient's feelings will increase.

How far should the expression of rage be taken? The obvious end point is the disappearance of the psychotic phenomena. It is a welcome sign when a patient turns and says, "Don't be so paranoid, Doc," suggesting that the patient is now the voice of reason. But I do not agree immediately; being older than most of my patients, I can say, "When you are as old as I am, you'll know how destructive some people can be." I want to explore as fully as possible the experience of the patient. Oddly, paranoid people tend to be ingenuous and forgiving. That may be one reason they become clinically paranoid: having trusted too far and then been double crossed, they still cannot locate the real source of trouble. I do not wish totally to allay their suspicions but, instead, direct those suspicions where the rest of us sensibly direct ours, to the world's real dangers.

It also appears often true that successful counterprojection produces depressed feelings. The beginning of depression offers a suitable finale for counterprojective efforts: when these efforts are continued into the patient's depression, they are received quite differently. The patient feels that he, rather than his enemies, is being attacked.

The same principles apply to the management of positive transference psychoses, that is, instances of excessive love for the therapist. A surprising number of therapists work by building love for themselves, with the goal of using it to motivate or control the patient. This is done in the name of a strong "working alliance." Of course, once having fostered love, the therapist may find that the patient has made some very extensive plans for his future. Many therapists, however, are able to make their patients fearful of openly expressing love, a subtle tyranny that forces the patient to love in secret. This may continue right through the rest of the patient's life, with a serious restriction of his capacity to invest elsewhere.

Therapists have difficulty expressing love for themselves. Politicians and salesmen find it easier. Therapists tend to be at least superficially modest and self-effacing, often to the point of spookishness. Speaking such words as "You must love me so much" is more or less the equivalent of standing on one's head. It is to be hoped that more therapists will interest themselves in making such empathic efforts, because they can marvelously deflate positive transference psychoses. They do not interfere with the patient's and therapist's appreciation of one another. Once the excessive love has been shared, and often relocated to old parental hopes, a real appreciation is likely to grow and be expressed. Most important, the patient may be freed from carrying a torch for the therapist far into the future.

There are at least two serious objections to the use of counterprojective statements. The first is the apparent encouragement they give to externalizing rage and blame, and the second is the danger of short-circuiting the patient's rage and therefore not fully working it through. Both objections are sensible.

It is unquestionably true that counterprojective statements encourage the externalization of rage. This can only be justified if such an encouragement is either necessary for emergency purposes or is at least partly true; that is, if external forces have been destructive and are to blame. The emergency justification can be supported simply on the basis of clinicians' sometimes needing to work within the patient's defenses—to begin where the patient is. This tactic should then be abandoned as soon as it threatens to distort the patient's realistic perceptions.

Because each of the principal schools puts responsibility for psychopathology in a different place, each regards social or contextual responsibility with differing enthusiasm. Orthodox psychoanalysis is often as derisive as biological psychiatry, since the main thrust of Freud's thinking was toward an intrapsychic and developmental etiology. Indeed, projection and externalization are seen as primitive defensive processes by which individuals escape their basic responsibility for psychic phenomena; psychoanalysis is an austere system of what is called rugged individualism in the economic sphere. Much of the Kleinian system is also unsympathetic to environmental responsibility. Externalization can be seen as "splitting" with the bad outside and the good inside, resulting in the paranoid position. Only social psychiatry regularly encourages externalization, because it sees pathological phenomena as a function of forces that are in part external. There are "pathogenic others" who can drive us mad.

It must be clear by now that I do not regard any of these points of view as adequate. Each is only a partial and possible solution to any psychopathological mystery. Psychiatry, like general medicine, should recognize many pathological loci and treat its rich material in an evenhanded way. In such a broad system, counterprojective encouragement of externalization is merely a hypothetical expedient by which one possibility of pathological location is explored. The psychiatric clinician is no more committed to it as a final truth than the surgeon is to appendicitis. Like the surgeon, the psychiatrist may change his mind once inside the patient.

The second objection to counterprojective statements nicely complements this pluralistic rejoinder. By externalizing and decreasing rage, therapists may prevent patients' "working through" and taking responsibility for their hostile feelings. It is even suggested that interpretations perform a vital function by mobilizing rage. A full-bodied therapy, it is contended, includes arguments and confrontations; too much empathy, kindliness, or deflection of rage will emasculate the work.

Furthermore, those therapists who see rage not as a reaction to deprivation or frustration but as the expression of a basic human instinct, perhaps Thanatos itself, want that rage harnessed. This is the purpose of taking responsibility for one's feelings. In such a view, therapists are never responsible for the rage of their patients, even when therapy is most frustrating, or even outrageous, because destructiveness is an instinct. If the therapist provokes that instinct, he is only bringing it to the patient's consciousness for the purpose of getting it under control.

This very Freudian argument has power and a beautiful cogency. But I myself do not know whether destructiveness is a reaction or an instinct, and I sometimes envy but cannot admire those who "know." Moreover, what seems to be decisive in the selection of tools is this very matter of control. We need to mobilize the fullest range and depth of feelings while still controlling those psychotic reactions that have baleful consequences. Interpretative methods have an unimpressive record in preserving that control. In contrast, counterprojection appears to succeed. Nor does it achieve that control by concealing or avoiding rage and love. Counterprojective statements are empathic precisely because they involve the expression of the patient's strongest feelings.

Gaining Perspective

Psychotherapeutic work is often conceptualized as a moving between a distant position and a close position, and of having the goals of both objectivity and intimacy.[10] Working empathically provides an opportunity for gradually building or increasing the empathic function in patients who lack it, for building a comfortable closeness toward oneself and others. Projective and counterprojective statements provide an equally important opportunity to gain perspective on historical experience and on emotional investments that have been carried over into contemporary experience as projections. In short, to lift the shadows.

The lack of empathy toward some aspect of oneself suggests distance between the judged and judging psychic parts. In psychosis, the critical part may even be experienced at a considerable distance from the patient, as in the paranoid hallucinations already mentioned. Finding empathy with oneself can be represented as a gain of psychological closeness between psychic parts. In contrast, gaining distance or perspective indicates a movement away from identification with some psychic part; some hitherto unconscious part of the person is then "seen" by the person himself.

Both these contrasting alterations in internal dynamics offer themselves as goals in equally contrasting clinical situations. Narcissistic patients, and many psychotic ones, are at a great distance from others and often from themselves. Their incapacity to enter relationships, see another's point of view, or form a transference neurosis blocks therapeutic efforts. Not until their empathic resources have been extended, as by the cultivation and maturation of what Kohut has termed the narcissistic or self-object transferences, is a collaborative effort of analytic interpretation possible. It is to this process that the development of empathic language makes a contribution.

Yet the difficulties that many other patients, and sometimes the narcissistic ones as well, bring into treatment occur not from a lack of transferences, or from their flat, indifferent, affectless relationships, but from their premature, even volcanic transferences and projections. Here the need is not transference cultivation, but transference management. Patients experiencing overwhelming transferences love and hate intensely and are capable of switching abruptly from one emotion to the other. They experience the present as something new, distinct, and unique. No matter how surprised, angry, or excited by present events they may be, though, it is really an emotion rooted in past events. The observer experiences surprise that they can still be surprised.

Similarly, however much pain is experienced, it is seldom felt symptomatically. Just as these patients have little distance from their pasts, so do they have little distance from their internal torments and little perspective on their characters. It is the world, particularly the present world, that is likely to be seen as symptomatic.[11] This does not mean that such patients have large empathic resources, but what they seem to lack most is inner distance, a perspective on their pasts and themselves. Empathy may even be clinically dangerous at an early stage, leading to heightened excitement and hopes. It is in the absense of perspective that projective and counterprojective statements seem most helpful.

Sometimes by confronting these patients with interpretations, particularly of the transferences, perspective can be achieved. Otto Kernberg has been the foremost advocate of this approach. Too often, however, they are enraged and become more paranoid. Kernberg himself has emphasized that a hospital or some other controlling structure needs to be close at hand. The first advantage of counterprojective work is the reduction of transferences to manageable proportions at relatively little risk. I have remarked that this is one reason why psychoanalytic therapy of children makes use of play objects. The objects provide a focus not only for the child's remembering but for his projections as well, thus reducing the projections on the therapist to a manageable level. Simultaneously, something enduring may be begun. This can be termed a "learning perspective," a differentiation of inner agencies, or a gaining of distance on introjected parts of the self.

This learning perspective is not an automatic result of working away from the patient; nor does the distance from the screen "out there" automatically become part of the patient's inner distance. Rather than being an automatic result, learning perspective follows from opportunities that the outer screen provides. Working on the screen means to concretely address, face, or look at hitherto undifferentiated parts of the self. These are not talked about or shared. Just as artistic perspective depends on such pictorial details as the size of objects, their separating distances, shades, and shadows, the color modulations that Cézanne exploited, so perspective in psychology depends on historical details. Perspective results from seeing things at once and in relationship to one another. A similar concept has been suggested by Samuel Novey, who found that gaining distance on the past was facilitated by visits to actual scenes of past events.[12] This is not always possible, of course, and much more often patient and therapist must paint the picture instead. Sullivan spoke of reconstructing the past as "what I would have seen if I had been there."[13] Writers also speak of "putting their pasts behind them" in the course of composing their autobiographies.

In addition, there is a likelihood that the gaining of perspective is assisted by its being shared with someone from whom projections have been lifted, at least for a while.[14] At such moments there is a unique present; the past is not falling on the other person. Perhaps this provides the sharpest perspective of all.

In summary, seeing by way of the shadows has some notable advantages. Narrative flow can be stimulated because projections do not fall so heavily on either patient or therapist, and some difficult clinical situations are relieved. A basic strength can also be cultivated in this way: perspective on the past, differentiation of the structures internalized in the past, and, above all, freedom from the past.

Performative Language

Tell a child he has told a lie, but never call him a liar, because that diminishes the sense of one's self.

Ideals and the Self

Finding fragments of the other and managing invasive projections, even the maintenance of a sound working distance between therapist and patient, do not ensure that the patient in question now attains a viable human existence. This is because the fierceness of critics, both internal and external, may make independent expression impossible. Psychotherapeutic means have to be found to defend the self. The principal device is the use of performatives.

Performatives are statements that perform an action simply by being spoken. The obvious contrast is to imperatives, which perform by making another person act, as in the psychoanalytic imperative, "Say whatever comes to mind." The concept of performatives is the work of J. L. Austin.[1] Here are his first examples:

'I do (sc. take this woman to be my lawful wedded wife)'—as uttered in the course of the marriage ceremony.
'I name this ship the *Queen Elizabeth*'—as uttered when smashing the bottle against the stem.
'I give and bequeath my watch to my brother'—as occurring in a will.
'I bet you sixpence it will rain tomorrow.' (p. 5)

Austin wrote that such statements "do not 'describe' or 'report' or constate anything at all, are not 'true or false'; and the uttering of the sentence is, or is a part of, the doing of an action, which again would not *normally* be described as, or as 'just', saying something."

Statements of appraisal and admiration may also be performative in certain circumstances. They bring into being the state of being appraised and admired. Of course, saying something does not always make it so.

> Speaking generally, it is always necessary that the *circumstances* in which the words are uttered should be in some way, or ways, *appropriate,* and it is very commonly necessary that either the speaker himself or other persons should *also* perform certain *other* actions, whether 'physical' or 'mental' actions or even acts of uttering further words. Thus, for naming the ship, it is essential that I should be the person appointed to name her . . . (p. 8)

Austin lists the necessary conditions. There must be an accepted conventional procedure that has a certain conventional effect. The persons involved in any particular case must be the appropriate ones for the invocation of the conventional procedure. The procedure must be executed both correctly and completely. The conventional procedures are often designed for use by people with certain thoughts and feelings, for example, the wish to unite with someone in matrimony or the thought of fulfilling certain promises or bets. It is therefore important to possess those wishes and intentions and, furthermore, to act subsequently as intended. These issues of sincerity and follow-through have particular importance for psychotherapeutic performatives.

These circumstances are easily applied to medical procedures. For example, operative and diagnostic procedures have agreed-upon steps with anticipated results. There are also appropriate people involved in the procedures, namely doctors and patients. Moreover, it is generally wise to execute the procedures correctly and completely. Finally, the last two circumstances could involve the honesty and good will of the physician, on the one hand, and the patient's compliance—say his willingness to take the prescribed medicine—on the other. This is not to say that the effects of surgery or medicine are due to the doctor's utterances in these circumstances. That would be to omit the knife and the medicine. The doctor's utterances can be very important, as with the acts of diagnosis and prescription. It is when medicine moves largely into the verbal realm, as in psychotherapy, that such a comparison gains its full significance.

There are a variety of situations in which these conventional procedures can go amiss. For instance, there are extenuating circumstances, such as when a performative is uttered under duress. A statement of admiration would not be performative if it were exacted by a threat, that is, it would not produce the state of being admired. This is perhaps most dramatically evident in lovers' quarrels. It is also a commonplace of medical transactions. The doctor may not pronounce a correct diagnosis of cancer because he feels it would be too great a threat to the person's well-being. Instead he gives an incorrect diagnosis. This is not quite what is meant by a performative, since the diagnosis is true or false whether or not the doctor pronounces it. What is dependent on the pronouncement, however, is the state of being diagnosed as such-and-such.

There may be no procedure acceptable to both parties. For example, I may accept a code of honor that includes dueling. In contrast, you may shrug it off. Austin remarks that this disparity is exploited in the unhappy story of Don Quixote. In the medical example, the patient may not accept the expertise of the therapist or, more commonly, may severely limit that acceptance. Furthermore, the particular persons and circumstances in a given case may not be appropriate for the invocation of the particular procedure involved. Austin writes, "Examples here are legion. 'I appoint you,' said when you have already been appointed, or when someone else has been appointed, or when I am not entitled to appoint, or when you are a horse." The psychotherapeutic analogue is obvious. Perhaps I am not a real psychotherapist, or perhaps you do not accept me as such. Maybe you deny that there is any psychotherapeutic expertise: there are then no accepted psychotherapists at all.

There also are failures to execute the procedure correctly and completely. I have mentioned already addicts who bring in someone else's urine lest their continuing addiction be detected. Then there are instances in which the failing is with the physician. I still remember with great distress the time during my medical internship when I drained what I thought was lung fluid, only to find that I had entered the lining of the heart. Psychotherapeutic procedures can go just as awry. Therapists may feel they are empathic when they are not. Performative efforts may support something that is not really a part of the patient, perhaps a quality projected by the therapist on the patient. The analogy to healthy and diseased tissue is again useful. The therapist, like the surgeon, must decide what is really the patient and what may be more or less a foreign object or a cancer.

The fault may also be on the receiver's part. For example, a promise may not be heard or understood as such. The same can be said about statements of admiration; they must be heard, even if it is with disbelief. This issue is of particular interest to the psychotherapist. Usually a performative of admiration will not be necessary if it is already fully believed. It should be used where it is at least partly disbelieved, even actively scorned. Yet it must be received. Special precautions are taken in law to avoid this mistake, one instance being the serving of writs and summonses. It has to be guaranteed that the person being summoned in fact sees the summons.

The idea of completeness or incompleteness of performatives can also be illustrated by statements of admiration. Consider the therapist who attempts to defend and develop in his patient some quality that is under heavy internal attack. If the therapist prematurely quits his effort, the development of that quality may stop or recede. The performative effort is essentially a contest between the therapist and someone else. Such qualities in the therapist as spirit and endurance are therefore crucial. There are also failures that concern the inner state of the participants. Do they mean it? Austin gives examples of not feeling what is pronounced: " 'I congratulate you,' said when I did not feel at all pleased, perhaps even was annoyed. 'I condole with you,' said when I did not really sympathize with you." The act is performed and not voided, as in many of the other failures, but it is insincere.

Must therapists always mean what they say, even feel what they say? Far from it. Projective statements, for example, are essentially hypothetical, playful. Sincerity is not the point. The point is to be evocative and experimental. Quite the opposite is true for performatives. There, as Austin indicates, sincerity is important. In fact, one of the perils of performative statements is that they may be very sincere but totally inaccurate. For example, many leaders impose on young people ideals at variance with their basic nature. I know a medical statesman with a following of loud, arrogant young people. Some of them are really that way; others only act the part, unreal people out of touch with themselves.

Psychotherapeutic Performatives

I have identified some useful performatives: appraising or reckoning, commending or admiring, hoping for, and wishing for. Each has an opposite or negative form that is sometimes more than "not appraising" or "not admiring," for example, condemning or cursing. Appraisals or reckonings are instances of what Austin calls verdictives. These "are typified by the giving of a verdict, as the name implies, by a jury, arbitrator, or umpire." An example is the umpire shouting "Out!" or the pathologist saying "That is healthy tissue." Appraisals or assessments of character, such as "I would call him industrious," also fit this category.

Psychotherapeutic verdictives gain their force from the expertise of the therapist. His appraisals may be wrong and may be subsequently corrected; they are frequently ignored. Yet they have special force in contrast to the psychological appraisals of umpires or even surgeons. This is most evident in the diagnosing process, but it runs throughout any contact with a therapist. It is one reason psychiatrists and psychologists are not always welcome socially; they are seen as specialists in appraising. It is like having an architect go through a beloved home.

By uttering the psychotherapeutic verdictive "You seem like

an industrious person" or the empathic "You must be lonely," a state of being appraised as industrious or lonely is created. A judgment or verdictive has been handed down, which is similar to the judgments of conscience and external authorities. Commending or admiring carries the idea of appraising into the area of value judgments. That is, a statement of admiration is both an appraisal and an appraisal of an appraisal. It says, "I like that quality." As Austin wrote, "here there is a special scope for insincerity." The performative of admiration is similar to the operation of ego ideal, as we shall see. While superego embodies the internal no, the ego ideal speaks the yes. These yeses range from simple acceptance, through admiration, to ideals and inspiration.

Note that the fact of the appraisal is separate from its force, whether from therapist or superego or ego ideal. Statements of condemnation or appraisal or admiration can have the force of the must: you must not or you must be, the so-called punitive superego or perfectionist ideal. These are important phenomena in the treatment of psychopathology. Therapists easily find themselves trapped in arguments with a patient's punitive or perfectionistic internal commands. If the therapist responds "You must" to "I must not," or "You must not" to impossible ideals, the patient becomes once more the battlefield of warring forces, and the ego is powerless to find its self. The performative of admiration is therefore not to be directed against the patient's internal agencies, but toward a beleaguered quality needing to be found and supported.

This is a distinction extraordinarily difficult to make with some patients. They are so allied with strongly critical internal forces that almost any statement to them becomes a fresh criticism. For example, a genuinely devoted and hardworking young female patient was subject to a virtually constant barrage of self-recrimination. She remarked that she could not recall ending a conversation without spending long periods in review of what seemed like her stupid remarks during the conversation. Often the content of the self-recrimination closely resembled comments her mother had made. It appeared that her mother, an editor for an academic press, always edited her children's utterances. The patient did not protest against these judgments of herself; in fact,

she sought them out by her meticulous reviews of her own conversations. The critical mental function or superego completely
controlled her value system; the patient was essentially supine.
One result was that the therapist's attempt to highlight this dependence and self-critical hegemony was seen as evidence of still
another failing. "You shouldn't be so self-critical" was added to
the list of her other inadequacies. This was not a trivial blow
because the patient felt that self-critical reviews of her behavior
were a strong point, that only by such means was she being kept
from a still worse fate.

For a period I was reduced to smiling at her, which, for all I
know, reinforced the self-critical behavior. The idea of performative statements was saving. The task became not to criticize her
for being self-critical, but to admire what she was generally critical
of. She accused herself of being garrulous, when actually her
comments were brisk and to the point; so I said as much. Very
gradually, this and other performatives created states of being
admired; the recriminations decreased. The process can be described as a balancing of critical superego with an admiring ego
ideal.

In my last chapter I discuss a patient whose tender and generous
impulses were under heavy attack from his masculine ideals; he
had come very close to homosexual panic. Through the use of
gradually more direct statements of admiration for these impulses,
it was possible to protect and develop them. This caused a state
of his being admired rather than condemned. Such a fostering of
what might be seen as femininity did not precipitate a homosexual
panic, for a reason that illuminates the nature of performative
statements, particularly in contrast to seductive ones. In essence,
by creating the state of being admired for a previously unacceptable quality, the patient's fear of homosexuality was dimin-
ished. This is because his fears arose from the condemnatory
machismo ideal; when that ideal was partly replaced by a different
one, the patient had that much less reason to fear. But a seductive
statement might have caused panic, since it could stimulate his
homosexual interest while doing nothing to offset the machismo
ideal.

Bringing about a state in which the patient has support in what he wishes or hopes for operates in a similar way. The statement "Oh, I wish you had that opportunity" expresses the desire for a goal or an ideal. "Would that you had . . ." indicates the same thing. An ideal is thereby shared, or a timid ideal is given robust expression and permission. The matter of being deserving is implied. In different words, it offsets the influence of any internal or external criticizing of a person's right to have such ideals.

"I hope there is someone who will put their arms around you" operates in a similar but more complex way. A lonely, wounded person might tempt the therapist literally to embrace the patient, a hazardous action best avoided. Yet the need remains. It is impressive that the expression of this hope for the patient acknowledges the need, keeps action out in the world where it largely belongs, and validates a sensible ideal. At the same time, it offsets any inhibitions the patient may have about his passive longings. Occasionally it achieves something still more important. A significant portion of humankind does not feel the right to hope at all—the future for them is absent. When a therapist expresses a wish or a hope, a little piece of the future is admitted. This is done performatively: the state of being hoped for is created.

Negative hopes can also be useful: they function as warnings. "I hope he's not like the last one," said to a hopeful lover who is not optimally discriminating, establishes the state of having been warned. Being negative, it partakes of superego additions rather than ones of ego ideal. It is therefore best reserved for the very hopeful. In the case of most of the remaining patients, superego additions from therapists occur only too readily.[2]

Managing Wounded Expectations

Jonathan, a handsome young man, much treasured as a child, found college competitive and joyless. As he remarked, he could not pack up his highschool reputation and take it with him. He sought help because of sleeplessness and fatigue, and I saw him later in consultation. The technical difficulty was to restore equilibrium to a proud man who disdained the casual approval of others. There was the additional difficulty of doing the restoration in a way that would not be so comfortable for the patient that, once again, he would not prepare himself for the future.

Jonathan had the look of someone who has been much looked at, and not with scorn or derision. The level of admiration he had become accustomed to before college was not likely to continue in psychotherapy either, so the work faced formidable obstacles. The first and perhaps most difficult step was to offset those great expectations, while simultaneously acknowledging and even honoring them. He needed to feel admired and to believe that his old purposes would not be totally abandoned, but at the same time there should be no foolish and impossible restoration of the status quo. Ideally, I would position myself for the defense of his expectations, while he carried the burden of self-critical appraisal. The patient should be warning *me* about the dangers of excessive hope. In this way I could stand with his former ideals, the loss of which depressed him, as he moved into the future. The patient could be the leader he needed and was perhaps suited to be.

Jonathan: Part of the process of therapy is just testing the expectations and finding out which aren't really realistic in the first place, and which would be true, which should be sacrificed . . .
Havens: You don't want to give up all your expectations.
J: No, but if I have no expectations, then I wouldn't do it.
H: One is supposed to need a certain amount of grandeur, right? [This is a projective statement. It could have been expressed proverbially.]
J: Well, I think actually many of my difficulties stem from excess of grandeur. I'm very hard on myself and I expect to be an historical personage.

This seemed to me a critical moment. It would be easy to diagnose narcissism and megalomania, with little appreciation of the motivating role these qualities can play. So I replied:

H: Maybe you can be, maybe you can be. That's a good idea. At least we need the right kind of historical personage, particularly right now.

He stuttered a modest protest, hardly a moment later acknowledging that he would not "resist" such a call to eminence. Then he stated the main point: he had been disappointed in his great expectations. Time seemed to be running out. He had wanted to be an "overnight sensation."

This could be more revealing than our relationship was ready to bear, so I diverted him toward intellectual matters while quietly urging a more generous attitude toward himself and the taking of time. It was necessary to avoid joining his self-accusations. It might even be advantageous to put off finding one's goals lest they prove false. In part this was a probe, using my reassurance to find the extent of his anxiety. The patient did not become complacent:

J: . . . and I sort of feel it's a fairly common dream, especially for people that are involved in performance, that you know they're up there on the stage, and the entire audience is looking at them with rapt attention, but they've forgotten their lines and they don't know what to do next, and for my next trick I'm going to . . . you know . . . there's no props or anything.

There was an audience he had to satisfy, probably a demanding audience, so I said straightforwardly, "It would be great to have something that you love." I wanted to support his wishes against those of the "audience." At the same time, I knew his wishes were still poorly formulated and not very specific. I had to be willing to settle for "inklings" at this time in his life. He then acknowledged there were some, but proceeded to underline the danger and pain of commitment:

J: Maybe you're a great painter, but if you never pick up a brush, then you know . . . and at the same time, it requires a certain amount of energy and effort to be able to say, "Well, I'm going to find out if I'm a good painter," and pick up a brush and start painting. Especially to find out that you're a terrible painter.

Even that might be tolerable, he said, if you were doing "something you love." Yet he did not sound convinced. We had entered a different part of the interview, in which the subject was *others'* expectations of him. Perhaps those expectations could be discussed in a relatively undistorted way, because I had been at pains to honor his hopes without being impatient for them. This was preventive counterprojection. I said, "Someone may have decided early on that you were gifted." Yes, and that once had its benefits; having a good reputation smoothed the way. Jonathan went on, "They gave you at least the benefit of the doubt . . . they fulfilled their own prophecies."

I did not pick up the "doubt." Was he really gifted or just the victim of what was almost a hoax? He was not yet on substantial enough ground, either in his life or in the interview, to approach that. Furthermore, it could only be a subject for fruitless rumination, which he had doubtless given it. The extent of his talents was something to be tested and established only in the ongoing opportunities of life.

H: Of course, being in that situation, although it would be lucky in some respects, it might be very unlucky if you then moved into a very critical . . . for one reason or another they didn't.

J: I think that's what happened to me. Was that, really, I wasn't able to sort of pack up my reputation and take it off to college with me. And it was really disarming, shocking even, to find that what formerly had been so easy, you know, the business of school work, doing the work and getting good results, had suddenly become extremely difficult, and I was no longer getting what I had come to think of as my due—approval, recognition. Really having opportunities offered to me. And instead of being the sought after and, I guess, valued, treasured, I was now just another guy named Joe, and it's hard to adapt to.

Here was a second crisis in the interview. He had again exposed himself broadly, rendered himself vulnerable to the judgment that he should not be so valued, should be only "another guy named Joe." Indeed, he almost brought that charge against himself. I know he did not mean it when he immediately laughed and said: "I think a lot of the democratic aspirations come from making sure that the other guy doesn't get an entree."

At such a vulnerable point it is essential to protect the patient's self-esteem. If his self-esteem is still more threatened he will almost certainly either retreat from the therapist or go on the attack. Jonathan had also given me a nice point of admiration in his ironical comment on democracy, his sense of humor. By admiring this I could help him endure the immediate danger to his self-esteem, as I substituted a realistic point of admiration for his "grandeur." (I could just as well have admired his psychological acuity.) That I accomplished at least this much is suggested by his deepening the confession of damage.

H: It makes a lot of sense. I mean, you appear to have weathered this shock. You haven't lost your sense of humor.

J: No, I've kept my sense of humor. I think it's become maybe a little more bitter, but one of the hardest things about . . . rather than any psychological problems is that it's internal damage. It's not always apparent, even to yourself, that something's wrong, because you know it attracts all sorts of attention to itself. But a lot of, when it's a psychological hurt . . . there is, I think . . . there's a difficulty, in the first place, of recognizing that there is self hurt, because there's an attitude of keeping a stiff upper lip.

He proceeded to elaborate the problem of "internal damage." First, there was the tendency to denial (physical treatments sometimes lessen the pain while exacerbating the underlying lesion); he pointed to the tendency of many other people to join in the denial, wishing him to keep his damage "internal." Finally, he mentioned that the problem became cyclical: fear of trying again kept him from restoring his self-confidence, which, in turn, deepened the helplessness and insecurity. I wanted to know how far this process had gone, so I "went below": was he suicidal?

H: Combining that with what you said about being critical of yourself, you may be wondering, you know, whether you're worth having around at all. It's reached the point . . .

J: Yeah, it did actually.

Yet this, he said, was a "blessing in disguise." Despair had made him see "how far off the mark I really was." I, in turn, did not know whether he was denying again or had the worst of his despair behind him. I was confident, though, that his despair was still close and needed to be shared. There was also the opportunity this offered of simultaneously countering inhibitions about closeness that might have contributed to the cycle of despair and isolation:

H: Well, I hope somebody during this dark period was able to throw their arms around you. It was a painful time. [A performative followed by a simple empathic statement.]

Jonathan accepted the empathic statement first and then dealt with the performative. People had to be pushed away because he could no longer respect himself:

J: It has been painful. I mean, I think usually perhaps of people trying to compensate. It seems the problem is full of clusters, and as I've gotten more disappointed in myself, many have also been disappointed in other people who were disappointed in me for their lack of judgment. It's like the old Groucho Marx routine about not wanting to join any club that would have me as a member. It's sort of I can't respect anyone that would have any respect for me, because I'm so . . .

Gradually I felt myself being asked to give up too; I felt him actively drawing me into the hopelessness. So I drew back:

H: Well, but some of them should be pushed away. That may not be your cup of tea . . . jumping on top of you.

This was an interpersonal statement, distancing and at the same time sharing his irritation and aloofness. He was not to see me as jumping all over him either:

J: Certainly not [laughter]. But what's really nice is if you can find someone that's sort of going, when they put their arms around me and however hard you push away, that's how hard they squeeze back. It sort of says, "Well now, I understand that you aren't very satisfied with yourself, and even though you don't like you, I like you. And I like you even though you don't like you." And sort of deciding that you're willing to fight for it. It gets very complicated.

I suspect he was able to acknowledge or perhaps newly develop this aspiration, not only because I had earlier "performed" it but because I had just counterprojected any fear he might have had that I would move too close.

In fact, no one had kept their arms around him. It was heartening that Jonathan didn't whine about it; he suggested that he was perhaps the one who might not know how to love. However, like the issue of his gifts, real or purported, his capacity for loving would probably be better developed later rather than scrutinized now. So I put it aside. For one thing, there was no way to decide if he genuinely believed he could not love or was depreciating himself in his depressive mood.

The next performative was less ambitious:

H: Well, I hope you found some people, anyway, that were at least companionable over this period of time.
J: I have. I've been very fortunate in that regard, I think. The difficulty is in being satisfied, I guess, with companionability and, I mean in my case, however much I have, it seems I always want more. And so there's always the . . . I guess . . . the feeling that this much is good, but more is better.

He again sounded his theme of great and disappointed expectations. Furthermore, falling in love, like commitment to a career, was unsafe because love could be an illusion and expectations could again be disappointed. What should he do, give up his expectations, modify them, wait? Whatever his decision, he might well need the therapist with him in the deciding, particularly if he was to transform his present demand into a future aspiration.

H: You bring some harsh accusations against yourself. I don't know how justified they are, you know. You call yourself, to put it in the same language, you've accused yourself of a hunger for fame, you've accused yourself of hunger for love. Not that those are irreversible . . . but you also accused yourself of impatience . . . I don't know how fair you are in that regard.

He wanted to be great, to be able to love. These splendid aspirations were still partly expectations, but he had begun to put behind him a time when he had believed they were already realized. Would he be forbearing enough to realize them in fact? Certainly he was unsure. And this was no time to add to his self-accusations. The therapist could not make him forbearing. If the therapist "ordered" him to persevere, he would be both accusing him of impatience and not sharing the often unbearable pain of waiting. Instead, the therapist expressed hope for that strength, and in doing so he brought a state of being hoped and wished for to this once hopeless and unwishing man.

How poor the human mind would be without vanity! It resembles a well stocked and ever renewed ware-emporium that attracts buyers of every kind; they can find almost everything, provided they bring with them the right kind of money—admiration.

FRIEDRICH NIETZSCHE

Defending the Self

With movement of projections away from the therapist and the world, that is, with successful counterprojection, paranoid people often become depressed. At this point the patients seem to resent the very counterprojective statements they had earlier welcomed. I speculate that, having shared the hostile feelings, the therapist has reduced them and, withal, the need for projection; essentially, the ego is strengthened by empathy and can reclaim the projected object. The object is still actively on the offensive, but now from within—hence, the self-accusations. Whereas the patient can join the therapist in attacking the projection when it is outside, the patient resents the counterprojective attack when it is inside because of this renewed identification with the object.

This is a nice confirmation of the theory that hostile projections represent unbearable feelings or ideas that can no longer be contained by the personality and are therefore put outside. It might be said that the unbearable must be shared, if that did not suggest a happier transmission than the recipients of paranoid projections usually experience. Still the value of the term "shared" appears from a different direction. When hostile feelings are shared by a therapist, they appear to diminish and can then be borne.

It is also predictable that they do not disappear. Their reappearance within the patient signals their continuance and also indicates that this bearing or containing of the feelings means at least a partial acceptance; they are again the patient's own.

Many have participated in this conversation:

Daughter: My mother makes me feel bad, she's so critical.
Friend: You shouldn't see her.
Daughter: She *is* my mother. Sometimes I need her.
Friend: You should ignore what she says.
Daughter: I try to but I can't.

Further, the daughter finds that she too is overcritical both of others and of herself.

The Internal Critic

Karl Abraham and Freud suggested that the human capacity to harbor an internal critic has two sources.[1] In Freud's words, "It may well be that identification is the general condition under which the id will relinquish its objects."[2] Faced by the necessity of separating from an actual object, the mind is capable of retaining it as an imaginary object. Moreover, it is not simply the object that is retained but the relationship to it, the feelings about it, including the feelings the object may have had for the patient. If these feelings are hostile, they may be turned against the self. The self-esteem of the depressed person is therefore under attack from two directions. The patient feels no longer loved from outside, and in addition he cannot love himself because he now incorporates a partially hated and hating object.

In the viewpoint of social psychiatry the emphasis shifts to external relationships. The depressive patient has been too good, too self-sacrificing. Others have taken advantage of this goodness; they are predatory or abusive. The depressive patient continually helps to recreate a critical environment by his choice of friends and the inability to defend himself. It is startling how abusive many depressive patients' friends prove to be. And therapists readily fall under the same spell, interpreting the behavior of the patient in a way that perpetuates this critical environment. As a result, it is difficult to know what part of the internal criticism against the patient is a fixed phenomenon and what part is simply a reflection of the patient's continuing interpersonal experience.

The existential psychiatry of depression centers on the patient, but from the viewpoint of understanding his striving in the world, his intentions, as opposed to internal mechanisms and defenses. The melancholic, from the existential viewpoint, sees himself as setting an example, religiously embodying goodness in an evil world, being willing to sacrifice himself for the eventual triumph of goodness. The patient's efforts and self-beratings appear to arise from the evils of the world and self-assessments of his own failures and limitations.

Psychoanalysis developed the most systematic treatment of self-depreciation, based on the parallels between mourning and depression. The goal is to mourn the internal critic, so often discovered to be the surrogate of an ambivalently held lost object. In essence, the conflict is to be resolved by discharging one party to the dispute. The discharge takes place through a process of remembering the relationship and feeling what one remembers. The patient again likes himself when freed of the internal critic.

This goal is very difficult to achieve with many patients. My hypothesis is that those in question have been so ravaged by intrapsychic conflict, and are the scarred battlegrounds of so many conflicts between so many hostile objects, that the latter cannot be ejected without leaving the terrain virtually barren. These personalities are like many small countries, which have hardly existed apart from the invading armies. They are the supine, no longer in a state of conflict because they accept as deserved the rain of criticism that falls upon them. In the conceptualization of inter-personal theory, they are passive victims. From the existential viewpoint, they lack purposes of their own. Extending the metaphor of the epigraph from Nietzsche, they become stocked with garbage. With these personalities, it is necessary to help build a part of the self that is independent of the warring introjects, if only to assist in their ejection. Performatives are directed to the development of such an independent element. Plainly, this purpose is not at odds with the mourning of hostile introjects; I think it assists the mourning.

Paradoxically, the very judgment of the internal critic provides the basis for the critic's eventual discharge. This is because what the critic condemns often proves to be the growing point of the patient's independent self. Gregory, soon to be described, found his gentle kindness largely condemned by his superego, which seemed to be the voice of an arrogant uncle. My performative statement of a different, admiring judgment on the gentleness and generosity developed those qualities to a point where Gregory could value them as fresh ideals. The result was internal conflict; the patient was no longer supine. He was in a position to decide what he wanted to be. He might decide to discharge the critic; he might decide to discharge the therapist. In either case, the judgment would be his own.

In major respects, performative remarks are the opposite of counterprojective ones. While the latter are aimed at the projected figures, point away from the patient, and often express the patient's negative feelings about the projections, performative comments voice positive feelings toward the patient and are about some feature of the patient himself.

The Place of Ideals

The power of performatives is based on the therapist's authority and on the patient's need to be loved. Such statements evoke and then transform the need to be loved.[3] Performatives are then experienced as the nidus of fresh ideals.

The relation between ideals and the need to be loved provides the entry point for the therapist's authority. Humans experience themselves as lovable insofar as they meet various ideals of beauty, goodness, strength, or just being themselves. Depressed persons do not feel lovable precisely because their internal and external dialogues indicate that they have fallen short of ideals. Megalomanic people feel lovable only so long as they can delude themselves into believing that they already represent the ideal. Performatives bring out the need to be loved and shape it in an adjusted relationship to ideals: the depressed patient finds that he is loved, not hated, for what is real about himself. The megalomanic can be loved for what is real and not delusional. These objectives are achieved by creating a state of being admired that is both obtainable and real.

Freud's cure through love did not mean any happy result that might spring from the love of a therapist for his patient. Quite the reverse; Freud directed attention to the patient's need or drive to love the therapist. Here we explore the equally hazardous need to *be* loved, both by oneself and by others. The cure through love then has another significance, which depends upon the therapist's finding in the patient a quality that can be admired, hoped, or wished for. It is the "recognition of a promise."[4]

The relationship between the patient and his ideals or, in the language of psychoanalysis, the relationship between the ego ideal and the rest of the mental apparatus is to be changed in two ways. The undefended patient is essentially demoralized, both the object of hostile criticism and its unprotesting recipient. First, the supine patient needs to find something to believe in. Second, having something to believe in means there is already an attenuation of the hostile criticism, that is, the patient does not identify with a globally negative assessment. As a result, the two ways in which the relationship is changed between the patient and his ideals are complementary: the statement "A self is found compatible with ideals" is the other side of "Ideals are found that are at peace with this self."[5]

It is not immediately obvious why self and ideals should have such an intimate relationship. Certainly ideals or values are an important aspect of the personality. They monitor behavior, in the form of superego, and inspire and give purpose, in the form of ego ideal. Nevertheless, that elusive and inclusive something, the self, also refers to the rest of the personality, for example, the person's wishes. If "feeling lovable" seems always to suggest at least an amicable relation between self and ideals, then maybe ideals, while a necessary part of self, are not enough.

New insight is gained on the meaning of self and the place of ideals with these words of John W. Miller: "The ego finds itself in the superego."[6] The meaning of self is illuminated because the ego, Freud's executive function, is not yet seen to be itself (or a self) until it comes into relationship with ideals. In other words, the self is precisely what emerges from the appearance of personally held ideals. This is no verbal sleight-of-hand. Until people are more than just instinct-gratifying objects, the behavior of which is more or less modified by expediency, there will be no need for the idea of self. The idea of self comes from the effort to find a harmony or integration among strivings, purposes, wishes, and various ideals. The concept of ego is not by itself sufficient to generate a self, because it is a neutral executive; for the ego, one solution is as good as another, so long as satisfaction or pleasure is maximized. The superego and ego ideal are exactly those parts of the personality that are not neutral about the type of harmonizing or integrating solution. The self is found by the ego in the superego because one's self makes the particular, individual selection.

The need to be loved also reveals the import of self and ideals. Suppose the need to be loved is an instinct—at what object is this instinct directed? Surely, at any object able to provide the loving. What is it that this other object loves? Does it love the need to be loved, the body, the ego? Each of these, as well as other parts of the person, can be the object of love. Yet we hear the frequent protest, "I want to be loved for myself." The reason this does not seem to be a pathologically narcissistic request is best seen in conjunction with self-love.

Self-love and self-respect are the result of finding the self. One may love his body, or her strong ego, or simply the happiness of being loved. Whatever is loved or valued can become part of the ego ideal. We can define ourselves through our body or ego strength, or our passive longings, which then comprise the ego ideal. In this sense, the ego finds its self in the part of the superego termed ego ideal.[7] In terms of loving others, we can enjoy someone or something and still not enjoy ourselves, because that enjoyment may conflict with our values: enjoyment, self, and values must be compatible.

The Field of Performative Action

Performative speech helps the supine person in impressive ways. Performatives gain their power from the supine patient's frustrated need to be loved and from the therapist's authority. The patient's need welcomes the authority of the therapist. Yet what justifies this imposition of authority? We have seen that the field of performative action is notably occupied by priests, judges, and kings. Priests and judges utter that most fateful of performatives, "I pronounce you man and wife." Royalty still confers knighthoods and christens ships. These declarations are performative because their utterance by certain people in special circumstances brings about, solely by that utterance, the states alluded to. These are all authoritative utterances, binding because of "the authority vested in me." What authority do therapists possess? I suggest it concerns the natures of psychic health and sickness. Just as the surgeon excising cancerous tissue pronounces one part healthy and another sick, so the psychotherapist performs his excisions. The pathologist may correct the surgeon, often too late, but that is only a fresh performative. The point is that a surgeon is vested with authority to cut, on the basis of his trained discriminations.

That the field of the psychotherapist's performative authority is psychological well-being and sickness (and not the operating room or the baseball field) is most evident in negative performatives. When the therapist pronounces someone schizophrenic, that person then is schizophrenic for many practical purposes. Of course another therapist may claim that the patient is not schizophrenic and lift the weight of negative judgment. Again, that is only another performative. Here the importance of authority is obvious. Which therapist is the greater authority on schizophrenia? Naturally some therapists have more authority than others. This puts them at great risk, since they can more easily impose their ideals and condemnations. They also are "ideally" placed to exercise that authority on behalf of the patient's ideals. Yet, because all therapists are authorities on psychic health, they can affect ideals and the need to be loved. The therapist who finds something to admire in the patient creates the state of being admired. This links him to the need to be loved, and what the patient is admired for becomes a potential ideal.

How is the psychotherapist to judge the health of what he observes? Particularly in the light of this book's extended emphasis on keeping open and not deciding, how are therapists to perform? At first glance, performative speech may seem remote from empathic acceptance or interpersonal balancing and managing. Actually it is not. Empathy with a beleaguered part of the patient establishes its existence, and the interpersonal need to balance the critical power of others helps to protect that existence. Performative speech also serves the purposes of keeping open. A criticized part of the self is developed; another possibility of human existence is preserved, and the patient is that much freer to decide.

Children with athletic propensities who grow up in bookish homes must somewhere find support for their natural inclinations, either in the home or outside it. Many do not and discover themselves isolated and denigrated, not only in the home itself but eventually in their own heads. It is toward such natural propensities that performative statements reach.[8] With them we enlist the invasive power of the mind, in order to protect and foster the unprotected. Yet is everything within the patient to be protected? The internalized parents would not agree. Perhaps they were right: Johnny might be better off burying his baseball glove.

The therapeutic answer seems to be clear: bring the tissue up and look at it. Often it is not easy to decide. In the case of psychotherapy, the final decision is not the therapist's anyway; even the surgeon cedes that to the pathologist. The psychotherapist acts to give the patient the possibility of decision, thereby increasing his possibilities of fuller existence.

Becoming Lovable

Performative statements evoke and transform the need to be loved. The evocation springs from the capacity of the therapist to admire. The need to be loved is transformed, in turn, in regard to what satisfies it. Johnny's athletic talent is now admired; its development becomes an ideal, its exercise a pleasure; it is no longer trivial or debased. Johnny can now enjoy *himself*.

The same process is evident in the performative treatment of megalomanic delusions. In these cases we can see most clearly that the self is transformed only after the need to be loved is evoked and transformed. The megalomanic person loves himself on the basis of a delusional reconstruction. This is generally an unstable basis for being lovable because there is little social context for its affirmation. It is also a static conception of self, which provides no opportunity for the working toward completion that gives a concrete sense of the self's reality. Nevertheless, the therapist brings a local stability to the megalomanic person by admiring him, by finding something real in the present to admire.[9]

The admiration by the therapist is first necessary in order to engage the patient; the therapist joins the patient in his view of himself. The therapist is then admired as part of the patient's inflated self. The engagement is deepened by this mutual admiration (forming what Kohut called narcissistic or self-object transferences), but the patient has already taken a forward step because he is partly looking at someone else as a source of something outside himself. He is not everything great; there is also something great that is partly outside himself. This is the first step in going from "I am great" to "I can strive for something that is great," in the transformation of infantile self-centeredness into ego ideal. The building of actual ego ideal originates when the therapist finds a quality the development of which beckons as an ideal. The delusional can then gradually be abandoned for the real, or, better, the potential, because it provides a more stable source of being loved. In the meantime, the mutual admiration society is maintained, lest therapist and patient disengage while its basis is being transformed.

The transformation of the self begins only after these steps have been taken because the finding, and even the acceptance, of something real to admire in the patient does not yet represent a change of self. The self is not reshaped until there is a working toward an ideal. The individual must strive to realize his ideals. This is the process by which the person becomes different and admirable.

The Languages in Action

> *We work in the dark. We do what we can—we give what we have.*
> *Our doubt is our passion, and our passion is our task.*
>
> HENRY JAMES

The Languages in Action

The following material illustrates the definitions, theories, and modes of action discussed. Again, I hope the reader will forgive the crabbed jargon by which these theories and methods are designated. (Often the development of psychiatry seems chiefly the substitution of one mouth-filling set of terms for another.) The reader should also beware any implication that every case follows the order of interventions used here. Not only is the substantial overlap of interventions a commonplace, but the order varies from case to case. Interpersonal language dominated the early course of this treatment because of the invasive nature of the patient's presenting psychopathology. A withdrawn, absent patient would have required empathic and performative efforts first.

Gregory, twenty-eight years old, entered treatment because he felt persecuted and helpless.[1] He was unemployed and living on money from his parents and his girlfriend. The patient called his mother "crazy" and his father a "passive cripple." He said he had almost gone crazy two or three times himself and was passive as well. When I kept him waiting for five minutes before the second appointment, he got furious and threatened to hit me. I responded with, "No wonder. I'm obviously not helping you either, no more than anyone else seems to have." This was intended to be counterprojective, that is, to move his fury away from me.

Gregory described a boyhood characterized by promising athletic and academic starts that eventually came to nothing. His persistent complaint was that no one ever guided him or, when they began to, subsequently let him down. I had the impression that he was an arrogant, boastful youth who took instruction poorly and was very unpopular, despite his considerable promise. His fantasy life had the typical persecutory and grandiose elements of a paranoid personality. The family was wealthy and prominent in a large southern city. Gregory alternately dropped and derided the names of well-known people. He could not imagine himself happy unless famous and powerful, yet he was actually doing little except smoking pot and demanding sex from his girlfriend (a dietitian).

The first goal was to separate myself from his hostile projections and to ally myself with him in examining them. To this end I could assert with enthusiasm, as he was doing, that no one had been able to guide him adequately and that his considerable promise was being wasted; this was incontrovertible. I maintained this position steadily, sometimes vociferously. We managed to assemble a substantial catalogue of such disappointments and wastes. Over a ten-month period Gregory went from demanding hostility to gentle depression. With the appearance of the depressed state, he gradually resumed work on his musical career and joined a religious group. My psychotherapeutic approach shifted from being largely counterprojective to being empathic and performative. It is the latter, depressive period I will describe in detail. (We met twice weekly through the whole two-and-a-half-year treatment.)

This period consisted of two distinct segments, the first lasting eight months. Early in the initial segment, angry outbursts were followed by tears and regrets. Then for the remaining six months tears alternated with hypomanic denial and pseudo-cheerfulness; the overt theme was often disappointment with his parents. In the second segment, the tears had largely stopped and the disappointment with his parents was replaced by disappointment with himself. Gregory subjected himself to a barrage of self-criticism. Yet he moved to a room of his own, stopped using drugs, and found a woman friend toward whom he seemed considerate and helpful. He began to make friends in the religious group. The pseudo-cheerfulness retreated as he became more active. This second depressive segment lasted about ten months, moving very gradually into the final neurasthenic and more neurotic phases.

The two depressive periods can be delineated by the conflicts present and the psychological spheres in which they were experienced. In the first, Gregory felt unloved; he wanted love but was full of bitterness and rage. He experienced this conflict less intrapsychically than externally, between himself and his parents. Furthermore, he could still identify himself with the pseudo-cheerful big shot he would turn against in the second depressive segment.

The later quarrel was largely internal. He was subject to an almost unremitting self-criticism, which he associated with his mother's criticisms of him during his childhood. In addition, he criticized himself for the lying and faking he still occasionally slipped into, which he associated with an arrogant but appealing uncle. The part of him that deplored the lying seemed different from the largely automatic criticisms of the maternal superego; it resembled more a self that wished to identify with an ego ideal of not faking. As this self was emerging, relatively free of the old introjects, Gregory became more active and in seemingly productive directions.

At the end of the second depressive segment, still another change occurred. During a visit to his parents, Gregory felt what seemed like a new warmth from his mother, and he reacted to it with the old withdrawal and panic. On this visit the mother seemed to be talking about herself more objectively and had only a few "reveries" in which she confused herself with the patient along grandiose lines. He therefore felt he should not have withdrawn and berated himself anew for missing yet another opportunity for love. He had moved from a paranoid attitude to a depressive one and finally to a largely neurotic position, subject to fears he found irrational. In the last position, there were also strong neurasthenic elements: he often felt indolent or paralyzed.

From the family or interpersonal perspective, the patient had not previously separated enough from his often irrational mother. The father had assumed a passive stance, in order to keep peace in the house, which only helped the mother to victimize their son. From the existential perspective, the patient, when first met, was experiencing a largely hostile world, which he had to conquer or be crushed by. Upon finding an ally against this world who shared his perception of it, the fear of being crushed subsided and, with that, his belligerence. Still he felt helpless and had no hope of ever being loved or coming to terms with his hatred. He experienced this as a war between himself and his parents. It was both tragic and unavoidable; hence, perhaps, his tears.

The subsequent internalization of the conflict was felt as a double disappointment. Gregory could not satisfy the internal critic, so grandiose and impatient, and if he tried to be like that critic—boasting, lying, looking down on others—he disappointed his new ideals. He found himself caught between the two ideal structures. This hesitation was often coupled with neurasthenic symptoms.

The Wish to Be Loved and the Wish to Hate

In the initial depressive phase, the patient yearned to be loved but disliked himself all the more for wanting that. The personality he put forward to be loved was an important, well-connected person who was actually disdainful of love. The grandiose personality differed from the violent person he often found himself to be. The latter was associated with his mother who, he remembered, would suddenly slap him. It was not an appealing image, and he tended to project it onto others; for example, at first he felt I might hit him. In contrast to the grandiose personality, with which he identified, the violent one could be counterprojected. Indeed it appeared that, through counterprojecting this relation, he went from the angry to the depressive phase.

In the first depressive phase, my therapeutic stance was a mixture of decreasingly counterprojective, consistently empathic, and increasingly performative statements. Each component was directed at a particular psychological difficulty. Gregory lacked distance on the family warfare: this called for counterprojection. He still denied, by grandiose pretensions, the sadness and bankruptcy of his situation: this required empathy with the underlying sadness. Finally, he found nothing to admire in the actual person he encountered in himself: the something-to-be-admired had to be established performatively. The same succession can be described in terms of the defenses. The initial predepressive phase was dominated by projections, hence the counterprojective method. In the first depressive phase, denial and manic pseudo-cheerfulness were most evident, thus necessitating the use of an empathic alliance with the denied failure. The final phase was typified by depressive introjection and the need for performatives.

Note that a purely counterprojective stance would have left the therapist attacking introjects that the patient identified with: for instance, the grandiose one. That would have been, in effect, an attack on the patient himself. An equally inappropriate stance would have been a solely empathic one, which would place the therapist in identification with some part of the patient that was despised by another part, resulting in the therapist's being despised also. The "family warfare" was spoken of directly and objectively to Gregory and, on one occasion, to his father. This was counterprojective because it was an attempt to avoid becoming personally involved in the warfare, which was spoken of as occurring "out there." The goal was to give father and son some perspective or distance on their quarrel, in accord with the technique of Murray Bowen cited earlier. The results supported Bowen's claim that if one nontransferential or undistorted relationship can be established, family turmoil diminishes. Then I could work empathically; at that time Gregory's principal defense was denial. Sharing his sense of failure, that is, dividing or apportioning it between therapist and patient, made it possible to credit the disavowed.

Early in the first depressive phase, Gregory's stance of

cheerfulness would briefly collapse into angry or tearful outbursts, the first pointing backward to the earlier paranoid position and the tears indicating the candid expression of sadness to come. At this point, he seemed more complacent than sad, and he did almost nothing. His attitude was: someone will rescue me; I am a gifted person whose pretenses are justified by my gifts. Later we discovered how justified this expectation was, for women in particular had always been available to support him, as his father would now.

I attempted to empathize with the bankruptcy by such remarks as "How does one begin at the beginning?" said rhetorically, not inquiringly; "It isn't easy to be at square one"; and "No wonder you feel like dying." A fairly steady, almost murmured drumbeat of such comments provided a background to Gregory's bland optimism. Usually the pseudo-cheerfulness would fade during the hour. As he became more willing to acknowledge his failure, sadness emerged; it seemed that, insofar as I was able to stay with it, the sadness in turn lightened, perhaps because I took part of it on myself. For many months there were wavelike repetitions of this sequence: pseudo-cheerfulness, sadness, then a more realistic brightening. In order to test the bottom of the patient's mood, I would refer to the possible hopelessness, changelessness, and endlessness of his condition. His mood would deepen, but only for a moment; he did not really despair.

The prevailing state became sadness and, paradoxically, where pseudo-cheerfulness had meant inactivity, the sadness was accompanied by a sharp rise in activity. Not only did Gregory begin to work, he sought people out. This was not for sexual use, as before, but for talk, companionship, even in order to help them. It appeared that the fact of bankruptcy had penetrated his consciousness and he was attempting to remedy it. It would be easy to conclude that he was merely trying to please me, which no doubt contributed, but the striking clinical observation was the change in activity accompanying the altered mood.

It was also striking how each improvement in Gregory's life, such as moving to a new apartment, buying a musical instrument, giving a party, was accompanied by an increased need of me.

This took shape in flurries of telephone calls, whose contents were remarkably similar: "Should I do this? I'm frightened and uncertain. I can't seem to decide." My remarks also had steady uniformity: "How can you decide? This is a hard one. I'm glad you have to make the decision and not me. It is hard to start." The last thing I wanted was to decide for him; that would have encouraged the old dependence and inertia. I did want to be with him in the sadness and uncertainty. Gregory's sadness was also accompanied by a striking increase of self-criticism. It had, in psychopathological terms, a strong depressive coloring. The self-deprecation seemed fully acceptable to him at this time. He felt the charges leveled against him were deserved. Gradually, however, the introjective origin of the abuses emerged. By that point, the performative work was well under way, and the self was emerging from its dominance by the introjects. Gradually, too, the denial disappeared. One day I was startled to hear him saying, calmly and objectively, "I can't believe I'm such a washout," at a time when he had stopped being one. It was as if the denial had cleared to let him see himself as he had been.

Increasingly I called attention to such qualities as his generosity and gentleness, which were under heavy attack from his bombastic, macho ideal. At first cautiously, and then more openly, I approved of these qualities. I suggested that perhaps they were part of him, and maybe not the least wonderful part. With this, my attitude changed. During the largely empathic phase, what I have called the first depressive phase, I was dour and serious. I was trying to imagine what I would feel like to be bankrupt, or, in terms of his defenses, I was trying to outweigh or oppress his pesudo-cheerfulness. As Gregory became sadder, self-deprecating, more active and less denying, I became less dour and more interested. I was less centered on his denied state of mind and increasingly more attentive and admiring of *him*. We were then coming into the performative phase.

In the first depressive phase, the dominant conflict lay between the wish to be loved and the wish to hate. This was dealt with counterprojectively by gaining distance on the family war and thereby reducing the hate. It was also dealt with empathically by sharing Gregory's bankrupt plight and giving him someone to be with in that plight. Finally, a performative attack was started by speaking directly to what could be loved—his artistic ambitions and kindness, supporting those qualities in defiance of the inner critics. The performative statements implied, "I can be loved for the very qualities that part of me and others have despised; I do not need to hate myself."

The Conflict between Ideals

Gregory no longer externalized any part of the conflict. His parents were no longer hated or seen as enemies. But when the patient assumed responsibility for the critical function himself, the artistic efforts and acts of kindness that had won the therapist's support now seemed to invite fresh self-criticism.

What probably happened was this: the critical function, once projected on the parents, had been drawn into the self, where it reigned supreme. Like an army coming home from abroad, it was seen everywhere, overwhelming the civilian population and seeming to be the voice of the whole nation. Gradually, however, and with the support of the therapist, other elements were heard from; a conflict was set in motion between these elements and the hostile ones. For a considerable period the conflicting forces were equal, and he was largely paralyzed. Then he became active again. Just as much of his activity before this neurasthenic phase had been in the service of the old bombastic ideals—only then he was to overwhelm everyone with kindness—so after the neurasthenic phase, when the new ideals were in ascendance, his kindness and artistic efforts became their own rewards.

What part did the waning of the denial play? At first, the principal conflict had been between the bombast and the facts, between his hypomanic pseudo-cheerfulness and the reality of his situation. The result was that Gregory came to see himself as a washout. Unfortunately, what was a victory for reality was also a victory for the bombastic ideal, which now had all its hostile prophecies fulfilled: if one was not a king, even a fake king, one was nothing. Only with the appearance of the fresh ideals was this state slowly reversed.

There was a complex period early in the performative phase when the issue was self-reliance. Gregory's family urged self-reliance on him; he was to "take any job you can get," and a previous therapist had told him to "assume responsibility" for his conduct. This seemed to me a mistake; his development was arrested at an earlier point in life, when he needed to test the reliability of others. Indeed, this testing seemed the main thrust of his passive-dependent behavior. I neither opposed the demand nor attempted to satisfy it. It was imperative to avoid offering myself for another test of reliability; that could involve an escalating series of demands which were very likely to be disappointed. In contrast, I justified his demands in terms of his past disappointments and, at the same time, stood with him in lamenting the unlikelihood of their being fulfilled. I too would probably disappoint him. This was a complex communication embodying counterprojective, empathic, and performative elements. I separated myself from those on whom he had been allowed to settle his great expectations; do not, I implied, expect too much from me. Empathically, I tried to share his disappointment and his hitherto acted-out and unspoken yearnings to be cared for. Finally, rather than either oppose or gratify his wish to rely on others, I approved it. This was performative, standing against the counsel of the parents and parental remnants, and singling out a quality for approval. This was a step beyond empathic sharing of a state of mind. It was close to a defiant statement of support from one person to another.

The discovery of Gregory's tender impulses occurred largely by accident. They were certainly not obvious parts of the bombastic and self-important personality he first presented. It is true that as soon as the counterprojection was well under way, and strong depressive elements had appeared, there also appeared a softness about him. But this seemed more like resignation than gentleness, and what generosity he showed was, at first, more a product of self-depreciation than of any genuine appreciation of others. One day the girl he was living with forged a check and was caught. He appeared more upset than she, blamed himself because he spent most of her money, comforted her, and arranged for legal help. He did not reveal any of this immediately but instead began scolding himself for his sentimentality. This was not the usual line of his self-criticism and made me suspect he might have done something useful. Knowing that he associated sensitivity with weakness, I did not reveal my suspicions directly. What I did do was to describe goodheartedness as something not entirely despicable, a remark he ignored. Then I mentioned that he might occasionally have fallen victim to the temptation of goodheartedness himself, whereupon he described what had happened and bemoaned his weakness. Subsequently I referred to his goodheartedness with increasing enthusiasm, on the average of once or twice every week, using simple performative statements—going from "Not everyone disapproves of generosity" to the direct "How wonderful you were so kind!" Essentially these were statements of approval directed at such qualities as reliability and goodheartedness that were under internal attack. I also made complex performative remarks, that is, a remark approving the quality and at the same time taking a further attitude toward the quality. An example: "Can I stay with what I love?" said imitatively. Here a loving attitude was applauded—and a strong empathic coloring was contributed by the imitative form. I joined the patient, offering to help bear the pain of persisting.

Another type of complex performative was the dominant intervention of the neurasthenic phase. This was a second imitative comment, "What do I want?" Recall that the neurasthenic phase has been hypothesized as one of paralysis between opposing ideals. Saying "What do I want?" implies that I have a right to want and there is an "I" who does the wanting. Both these implications confronted Gregory's self-criticism.

The replacement of simple statements of approval with "What do I want?" also represented the therapist's retreat—I stepped back to let the patient decide between ideals. I did hope for a decision; that is also implied by the question. Yet I tried to meet each of the patient's arguments for one side of the debate by restating the arguments of the other. When Gregory spoke of wanting to use a woman sexually, I would respond, "Good luck. With your good heart you'll probably make a mess of it." When he asked, "Can I live without pretenses?" I asked, "Can anyone?" A review of my notes indicates that most of the arguments in this phase were for the old ideals. Gregory had now taken up the new ones so devotedly that I feared he would once again neglect a part of himself. But the stating of opposite positions was not so much for the sake of balancing considerations as of validating his need and right to decide. The very fact that I represented opposite sides and seemed, for the most part, to have adopted his old ideals, freed me from the charge of representing anything but him. It was to be his decision, not mine. To impose my wishes would only replace one set of tyrants with another. In fact, he gave up "being great" to cultivate things in himself that could become great.

When I first met him, Gregory was a domineering personality, sometimes a frightening one. This outer domination was paralleled by an inner domination: he had to be the great figure he associated with his parents and uncle. At the same time, he experienced the outside world as dominating him. Even the hint of an antagonistic act by another was considered a violent attack, calling forth his own aggression in return. Domination and submission were the themes of Gregory's life: domination of the world but submission to the ideals of family, feared submission to the attacks of others, domination to counter them. Where was he in all this warfare? He was hardly present in the megalomania, so easily punctured, so little deceiving even himself. Nor could he be present in submission. The result was largely faceless absence or an existence careening back and forth between the two poles.

I engaged this patient by an acknowledgment, rivaling him in vociferousness, that indeed no one had helped him. This shared his fury. But implicit was an element surfacing much later as an outright performative: my implying that there was or could be someone present who *should* be helped. It is not enough to say that this is always part of the contract between therapist and patient. The fact is, it must be felt by the patient. I made it felt by the vehemence of my sharing in his rage. There was really something to be mad about: the loss of such a person. In this sense all my utterances were implicitly performative, conveying that there was the possibility of a person to be found or developed.

I close on this note because this book's concern with theory and language should not obscure the place of passion. Caring is the term most often used for clinical concern, but the word passion better transmits the deep-running sense of interest and often outrage that must infuse difficult and persistent clinical efforts. Of course this has to be a disciplined passion. The emphasis on language and theory given here is no more than the form of that discipline, the engineering structure necessary to translate passion into what is clinically effective. Nor can that passion often risk showing itself. As with the great stresses that engineers must mobilize and control, effective clinical behavior needs to render the presence of passion largely invisible, like the still structure of a bridge. The danger of making therapeutic concern explicit is that some patients misunderstand. As I have said, many are not helped by knowing we care; they are only made more passive and hoping. Others will see any interest as exciting or seductive. Even more important, the energy of concern needs to be conserved for effective action; it cannot afford to waste itself in empty display. It is by its results that therapeutic passion is best known.

In this way psychotherapy transcends explaining and talking things over with patients—too often an intellectual exercise. In reaching disciplined passion, psychotherapy becomes an activity calling on shrewd intuition and the strenuous use of feeling and control. What the therapist can translate into effective action the patient can use to construct a livable existence.

Notes

Acknowledgments

Index

Notes

Finding the Other

1. George E. Vaillant, "Sociopathy as a Human Process," *Archives of General Psychiatry,* 32:178 (1975).

2. See Orlando Patterson, *Slavery and Social Death* (Cambridge: Harvard University Press, 1982).

3. This was pointed out to me by Daniel Lowenstein, who was then a third-year medical student at Harvard.

4. J.-M. Charcot, *Clinical Lectures on Certain Diseases of the Nervous System,* tr. E. P. Hurd (Detroit: Davis, 1888), lecture 7.

5. Pierre Janet, *The Major Symptoms of Hysteria* (New York: Macmillan, 1907).

6. H. F. Ellenberger, *The Discovery of the Unconscious* (New York: Basic Books, 1970), p. 98.

7. Empathy is also the projection of one's mental state onto another person or object. This is empathy from the viewpoint of the sender. There is always the problem that what seems like the therapist's receipt of another's mental experience is really the therapist's transmission of his own. Psychoanalytic work suffers from the same difficulty of separating transference and countertransference.

8. Martin Buber, "Elements of the Interhuman," *Psychiatry,* 20:110 (1957).

9. Eugen Bleuler, *Dementia Praecox, or the Group of Schizophrenias* (New York: International Universities Press, 1959), p. 455.

10. It has been claimed to be the most reliable sign of schizophrenia: G. Irl, "Das 'Praecoxgefuhl' in der Diagnostic der Schizophrenie," *Archiv für Psychiatrie,* 203:385–406 (1952). But so have many other phenomena.

11. Bleuler wrote of changes in "affective rapport" (*Textbook of Psychiatry,* New York: Macmillan, 1930, esp. pp. 438 and 525), and E. E. Southard, of the empathic index ("The Empathic Index in the Diagnosis of Mental Diseases," *Journal of Abnormal Psychology,* October 1908). For a general review of the literature, see Harry Wiener, "External Chemical Messengers, I and III," *New York State Journal of Medicine,* 66 and 67:3153, 1287–1310 (1966 and 1967).

12. Sociologists have conceptualized these phenomena as owing to: social facilitation (F. H. Allport, *Social Psychology,* Boston: Houghton Mifflin, 1929); rapport (R. E. Park and E. W. Burgess, *Introduction to the Science of Sociology,* Chicago: University of Chicago Press, 1921); circular reactions (N. E. Miller and John Dollard, *Social Learning and Limitations,* New Haven: Yale University Press, 1941); and contagion (G. LeBon, *The Crowd,* New York: Viking Press, 1960; 1st ed. 1895). For more recently observed phenomena, see *Mass Psychogenic Illness: A Social-Psychological Analysis,* M. J. Colligian, W. Pennebaker, and L. A. Murphy, eds. (Hillsdale, N.J.: Ehrlbaum, 1982). In this, the understanding is more cognitive than affective.

13. Edmund Husserl, quoted in Rollo May, Ernest Angel, and Henri F. Ellenberger, eds., *Existence: A New Dimension in Psychiatry and Psychology* (New York: Basic Books, 1958), p. 76.

14. Ibid., p. 37.

15. Eugene Minkowski, *Lived Time: Phenomenological and Psychological Studies,* tr. Nancy Metzel (Evanston: Northwestern University Press, 1970).

16. F. T. Melges, *Time and the Inner Future* (New York: Wiley, 1982).

17. Ludwig Binswanger and the psychoanalyst Hans Leowald come to a very similar conclusion.

18. Alfred Stanton, "The Significance of Ego Interpretive States in Insight-Directed Psychotherapy," paper delivered at the Boston Psychoanalytic Society and Institute Memorial Symposium for Elvin V. Semrad, November 18, 1977. For a further discussion of these categories, see Karl Jaspers, *General Psychopathology* (Chicago: Chicago Press, 1964), pp. 106–107.

19. From Cummings' poem, "Maggie and Millie and Mollie and May."

20. Einstein wrote in his autobiographical sketch: "No ever so inclusive collection of empirical facts can ever lead to the setting up of such complicated equations. A theory can be tested by experience, but there is no way from experience to the setting up of a theory." And in an earlier passage from the same work: "I see Mach's greatness in his incorruptible skepticism and independence; in my younger years, however, Mach's epistemological position also influenced me very greatly, a position which today appears to me to be essentially untenable. For he did not place in the correct light the essentially constructive and speculative nature of thought and more especially of scientific thought." *Albert Einstein: Philosopher-Scientist,* ed. P. A. Schilpp (London: Cambridge University Press, 1969), I, 89, 21.

Imitative Statements

1. Interest in the self waxes and wanes through the history of psychiatry. It was not a notion that attracted Freud, who preferred to study its elements and avoided the holistic introspectionist attitudes that are comfortable with it. Yet among the early Freudians there were some who felt the idea was important, notably Adler and Rank. Today there is great interest in the self, most prominently by Erikson, Lifton, and Kohut. It remains unattractive within the main body of psychoanalysis. The same is true for many Sullivanians, who maintain that the self is a social fiction. Currently we have no pathological schema of the self. It is easy to imagine constructing one from dictionary lists of compounds: self-effacing, self-abnegating, self-aggrandizing, self-centered, and so on.

2. Patients are given first names in my text for ease of reading. I don't use names in therapeutic work, and the identifications here are not an avowal of such use. Naming of patients to their face is powerful stuff. Use of first names suggests familiarity; it also can indicate a condescending or infantilizing attitude, especially if the therapist is not similarly addressed. Use of names also supposes, in the most immediate way, that there is someone present. This has to be established, not supposed.

3. Men and women have "the impression that the alien gaze which runs over his body is stealing it from him, or else, on the other hand, that the display of his body will deliver the other person up to him, defenseless, and that in this case the other will be reduced to servitude. Shame and immodesty, then, take their place in a dialectic of the self and the other which is that of a master and slave; insofar as I have a body, I may be reduced to the status of an object beneath the gaze of

another person, and no longer count as a person for him, or else I may become his master and, in my turn, look at *him*. But my value is recognized through the other's desire, he is no longer the person by whom I wished to be recognized, but a being fascinated, deprived of his freedom, and who therefore no longer counts in my eyes." Maurice Merleau-Ponty, *Phenomenology of Perception*, tr. Colin Smith (New York: Humanities Press, 1962), pp. 166–167.

4. To be naked is to wear one's heart on one's sleeve, in D. W. Winnicott's words. It is to be without a false self, which is for social functioning, or without a false personality, which is crippling. *The Maturational Processes and the Facilitating Environment* (New York: International Universities Press, 1965).

5. Quoted in John Updike's "Reflections," *The New Yorker*, May 9, 1983, p. 129.

6. Richard Ellmann tells the story of James Joyce's consultations with Carl Jung over his schizophrenic daughter, Lucia: "When the psychologist pointed out schizoid elements in poems Lucia had written, Joyce, remembering Jung's comments on *Ulysses*, insisted they were anticipations of a new literature, and said his daughter was an innovator not yet understood. Jung granted that some of her portmanteau words and neologisms were remarkable, but said they were random; she and her father, he commented later, were like two people going to the bottom of a river, one falling and the other diving." *James Joyce* (New York: Oxford University Press, 1982), p. 679.

Simple Empathic Statements

1. Harry S. Sullivan, *The Psychiatric Interview* (New York: Norton, 1954, 1970).

2. Charles Darwin, *The Expression of Emotion in Man and Animals* (Chicago: University of Chicago Press, 1965), pp. 163, 205.

3. "It is surprising how frequently the client uses the word 'impersonal' in describing the therapeutic relationship after the conclusion of therapy. This is obviously not intended to mean that the relationship was cold or disinterested. It appears to be the client's attempt to describe the unique experience in which the person of the counselor—the counselor as an evaluating, reacting person with needs of his own—is so clearly absent. In this sense it is impersonal . . . the whole relationship is composed of the self of the client, the counselor being depersonalized for the purposes of therapy into being 'the client's other self.'" Carl R.

Rogers, *Client-Centered Therapy* (Boston: Houghton Mifflin, 1951).

4. In what other way might the use of rhetoric be made palatable? Perhaps the professional reader should be reminded about an earlier generation which was appalled by Freud's speaking to patients of sexuality. In particular, Freud's warning might be cited—that by dealing with sexuality real dangers are conjured up that in some instances might prove unmanageable. One can emphasize his justification that powerful forces might be no less powerful for being ignored and, in fact, are best not left unheeded and unconscious. Doubtless the contemporary professional will be unmoved. He might reply that talk of private matters, emotional talk, is all very well for the patient but not for the professional. The reason the patient's emotions can be mastered is that the analyst's have been; he is rational, not rhetorical. It is only in the cool, serene light of rational discourse that the great forces Freud uncovered can be understood and controlled. I hope the limitations of cool verbal analysis are now well enough known to make the use of other devices appealing, especially in a therapeutic climate that is replete with permission to use powerful chemical and electrical interventions.

5. My interview material here is as accurate as my notes, which were written afterwards. It includes everything that occurred as well as I can remember, except where gaps are indicated. I do not vouch much for the accuracy of these recollections. The reader will often note a different tone when tapescripts are used, as in all the later illustrations.

Complex Empathic Statements

1. On the other hand, some workers, for example Henri Bergson (cited in G. W. Allport, *Personality: A Psychological Interpretation,* New York: Holt, 1937, pp. 530–553), regard empathy as the basis of intuition. I believe the critical point is where the observer places himself, whether to be with the other or himself, a projective or introspective stance. M. F. Shore has made a further distinction between what he calls self-effacing and self-involving empathy, depending on whether one attempts to put oneself aside and enter into the other's state of mind or to project oneself onto the other (personal communication, 1980). This is not the same as my passive and active empathy, both of which are self-effacing. Compare Freud's statement that empathy is necessary only with the unfamiliar. The implication is that with the familiar one can make reference to one's own experience, as by intuition.

2. Psychotic denial can be distinguished from the neurotic type. In

catatonic denial the feared person or event is obliterated, as in negative hallucinations. In manic denial the actuality is transformed into its opposite, poverty into wealth, etc. The feature that is most interesting about the neurotic or normal person's denial is the capacity to avoid being in the presence of fact and feeling at the same time. For example, the obsessional person can isolate feelings when discussing a difficult event or keep his mind blank when feeling something.

3. See Sullivan, *The Psychiatric Interview,* pp. 21–23.

4. Joseph Breuer and Sigmund Freud, *Studies on Hysteria* (Standard Edition), vol. 2 (London: Hogarth Press, 1955).

5. The importance to psychotherapy of such widely held ideals cannot be overstated. For example, the women's movement has been of immense value for psychotherapy because it has held out the ideal of women's freedom and equality to any woman struggling under difficult circumstances to assert herself. It therefore gives therapists a mode of entry to many domestic and work conflicts. The place of ideals in psychiatry will be further developed in the subsequent chapters.

6. Elvin Semrad encompassed much of psychotherapeutic work in his formula: acknowledge, bear, and put in perspective.

7. Bertram D. Lewin, *The Psychoanalysis of Elation* (New York: Norton, 1957).

Extensions

1. For a discussion of these phenomenological categories, see Jaspers, *General Psychopathology,* pp. 108, 117.

2. Elvin Semrad, personal communication, 1965.

3. L. L. Havens, "Placement and Movement of Hallucinations," *International Journal of Psychoanalysis,* 43:426–435 (1962).

Good Management

1. See H. F. Searles, "The Analyst's Participant Observation as Influenced by the Patient's Transference," *Contemporary Psychoanalysis,* 13:367–371 (1977). Searles has been the foremost student of this phenomenon. For example, he describes having felt almost moribund while working with one patient. He first attributed this to fatigue, since he had been working hard, but said that gradually "transference-material emerged which made it clear he was reacting to me variously as his chronically depressed mother, and as a long-senile grandmother who had lived

nearby, largely as a vegetable, during a considerable portion of his developmental years." Searles also referred to having been pleased by a favorite patient. For a period, this kept the patient pleasing the therapist and away from the long-experienced resentment' of having to please others.

2. Freud, *Recommendations to Physicians Practising Psycho-Analysis*, Standard Edition, vol. 12, pp. 111–112.

3. Alfred Margulies and Leston Havens, "The Initial Interview," *American Journal of Psychiatry*, 138:421–428 (1981).

4. A. Natapoff, "Evolution of the Human Brain," *Perspectives in Biology and Medicine*, Spring 1976.

Projective Statements

1. Originally I grouped projective, counterassumptive, and counterprojective statements under the concept of counterprojection, based on a study of Harry Stack Sullivan's interventions (*Participant Observation*, New York: Aronson, 1976). Joseph Glenmullen suggested the present terminology and also the substitution of counterparapraxis for the term I have continued to use, counterprojection.

2. W. S. McFeely, *Grant: A Biography* (New York: Norton, 1981).

3. I'm not sure modesty and authority are within the reach of beginners. Beginners feel only too acutely the fraudulence of their authority. Any procedure, such as making marks, that opens the way to or indeed welcomes mistakes will only increase the beginner's sense of vulnerability. How could someone be openhanded who feels, "Let the patient once know how ignorant I am and he'll run me out of the room"? This is what sets the agenda for those who supervise beginners. The latter need to borrow the authority of the supervisor. Lest that authority be too much borrowed, supervisors will seldom be wrong to remind beginners that there is more than one way to do the work.

4. Lytton Strachey, *Literary Essays* (New York: Harcourt Brace, 1949), p. 222.

5. Compare E. G. Mishler's work on language in the classroom: "the general hypothesis about the relationship of the linguistic structure of discourse to differentials between speakers in authority is examined through an analysis of natural conversations in first-grade classrooms. The findings provide consistent support for this hypothesis. When adults initiate a conversation with a question, they retain control over its course by successive questioning, i.e., by Chaining; when children ask an adult a

question, the adult regains control by responding with a question, i.e., by Arching. Children question each other through a more balanced use of Chaining and Arching that might be thought of as either more egalitarian, or more competitive." "Studies in Dialogue and Discourse: I. Types of discourse initiated by and sustained through questioning." *Journal of Psycholinguistic Research,* 4(2):99–121 (1975).

Counterassumptive Statements

1. People are expected to lose their "stranger anxiety" in the course of development. I'm not sure they do. Perhaps they learn to disguise it or, more likely, most people newly met do not seem strangers after some point in development. They are assumed to be like you and me. My point is that when people newly met *do* seem strange, as is true of many patients with very serious characterological problems, they provoke stranger anxiety.

2. May Sarton, personal communication, 1983.

Counterprojective Statements

1. D. W. Winnicott, *Therapeutic Consultations in Child Psychiatry* (New York: Basic Books, 1971).

2. A. T. Beck, "Cognitive Therapy: Nature and Relation to Behavior Therapy," *Behavior Therapy,* 1:184–200 (1970).

3. David Garfield, personal communication, 1982.

4. Fritz Perls, *The Gestalt Approach and Eyewitness to Therapy* (Palo Alto: Science and Behavior Books, 1973).

5. Murray Bowen, *Family Therapy in Clinical Practice* (New York: Aronson, 1978), pp. 308, 313–314.

6. Otto Kernberg, "The Treatment of Patients with Borderline Personality Organization," *International Journal of Psychoanalysis,* 49:600–619 (1968).

7. See Jay Haley, *Uncommon Therapy* (New York: Grune and Stratton, 1968); Richard Bandler and John Grinder, *The Structure of Magic,* vol. 1 (Palo Alto: Science and Behavior Books, 1975). Bandler and Grinder, as well as Haley, give examples of the occasional therapeutic *usefulness* of double-binding statements to highlight existing inner conflicts. It seems to me, however, that in their almost exclusive dependence on questions, these workers introduce many other, unintended, contradictions of medium and message.

8. Contradictions of medium and message can be thought of as inducing inner oppositions of insight-oriented and behavioristic models of learning.

9. To my knowledge, there is no accepted term for the second type of repetitive act, which depends on selection rather than misperception, in fact, on accurate perception of the selected objects. Enactment seems a good term, but this is already in the literature, with a broader meaning of any acting out of any unconscious process. Joseph Sandler, Christopher Dare, and Alex Holder, *The Patient and the Analyst* (New York: International Universities Press, 1973).

10. Dieter Wyss, *Psychoanalytic Schools from the Beginning to the Present* (New York: Aronson, 1973). See the last two pages.

11. Therefore, it is sometimes argued, patients need to take responsibility and not be encouraged to externalize further, as by counterprojection. But people cannot be forced to take responsibility; they will be responsible for what they are strong enough to take responsibility for. Counterprojection often increases both perceptiveness and the sense of strength.

12. Samuel Novey, *Second Look: The Reconstruction of Personal History in Psychiatry and Psychoanalysis* (Baltimore: Johns Hopkins University Press, 1968).

13. R. G. Kvarnes and G. H. Parloff, eds., *A Harry Stack Sullivan Case Seminar* (New York: Norton, 1976).

14. Everyone experiences the loss of perspective that results from excessive closeness, whether in looking at physical objects or in personal relationships. This is the reason that the doctor who treats himself has a fool for a patient.

Ideals and the Self

1. J. L. Austin, *How To Do Things with Words* (Cambridge: Harvard University Press, 1962, 1975). Before realizing the psychotherapeutic import of Austin's work, around 1978, I had been calling performative language "counterintrojective," at the suggestion of James Longcope.

2. On hearing this material presented, Gerald Adler (1983) remarked that when he and Leon Shapiro worked in the Massachusetts prison system, they often experienced the prisoners as inviting their therapists to take an actively negative view of the prisoners. It was necessary to oppose this temptation in a manner similar to performatives.

Defending the Self

1. Karl Abraham, *Selected Papers* (New York: Basic Books, 1957); manic-depressive states and the pregenital levels of the libido, pp. 418–501. Freud, *Mourning and Melancholia,* Standard Edition, vol. 14, pp. 243–258.

2. Freud, *The Ego and the Id,* Standard Edition, vol. 19, pp. 1–66.

3. The phrase is Barry Roth's, personal communication, 1979.

4. James Longcope, personal communication, 1978.

5. For evidence that morale and remoralization are central psychotherapeutic processes, see Jerome D. Frank, *Persuasion and Healing* (Baltimore: Johns Hopkins University Press, 1961).

6. J. W. Miller, *In Defense of the Psychological* (New York: Norton, 1983), p. 10.

7. Freud has often been criticized for turning instinct gratification into an ideal, for reducing humans to their animal appetites and justifying a hedonistic society. The criticism is not justified because no one was more exquisitely aware than Freud of the need for a balance of social constraints and individual gratification. The point of misunderstanding arose because he believed that neurotically repressed individuals were in need of ceding to gratification a greater place in their ideals.

8. The frequent occurrence of such inhibiting antagonisms in families is perhaps most often due to the genetic mixing that occurs in the human reproductive process. While this provides variety in the struggle for existence, it also causes trouble.

9. The first two of these three steps Kohut has called the idealizing transferences, which he sees as an especially paternal role in normal development. Heinz Kohut, *The Restoration of the Self* (New York: International Universities Press, 1977).

The Languages in Action

1. This case material was part of a paper Barry Roth and I presented at the William Alanson White conference on converging trends in psychoanalysis, January 25–27, 1980.

Acknowledgments

I have cited the contributions of many colleagues in the text and notes. A list of these colleagues must certainly include Alfred Margulies, James Gustafson, Jack Burke, Henry White, Doris Menzer-Benaron, Thomas Gutheil, David Mann, Harold Bursztajn, Barry Roth, David Garfield, and Joseph Glenmullen. Yet so many ideas that seem to arise in one's own head have really been put there or come from a collision of minds, as at home with Susan Miller-Havens or at lunch with my old and dear friends Myron Sharaf and Alan Natapoff, that no list could be complete.

I am greatly in the debt of Hilary Palmer, Nicole Jordan, and most notably Cal Kolbe, who typed and edited various stages of this manuscript. I also want to thank Harvard University Press for the incomparable Joyce Backman, and Arthur J. Rosenthal for his patience, enthusiasm, and a marshal's eye.

Different versions of some chapters in this book have appeared in *Contemporary Psychoanalysis*, the journal of the William Alanson White Psychoanalytic Society and the William Alanson White Institute; in *Psychiatry: Journal for the Study of Interpersonal Processes;* and in an audio program on interviewing techniques done for The McLean Facility for Continuing Education.

Index

Abraham, Karl, 160
Absence, forms of, 3
Actor, defenses of, 11–12
Adjectives, 43–44
Admiration, 144–147
Adult precipitants, and psychoses, 73
Affect, 17–19, 51, 89
Affective baseline, establishing, 48–49
Ambivalence, 38, 61
Antipathetic responses, 43
Anxiety, 86–87
Appraisal, 144, 147
Approximating elements of conflict, 71–78
Arguments, 136
Assumptions, shaking of, 111–123
Attention: and counterprojective statements, 126; and free response, 93; Freud on, 88–89, 90, 92; and projective statements, 125
Attitudes: in interpersonal and existential work, 91; signaling, 112–113
"Audience," vs. personal wishes, 152
Austin, J. L., 143–144, 145, 147
Authority: and ignorance, 102; imposition of, 165; patient's need for, 103; in psychotherapy, 85; therapist's burden of, 102–103

Beck, Aaron, 126
Bewilderment, 117, 118, 119, 120, 122
Blame, 135
Bowen, Murray, 127, 175
Bridging statements, 57, 59, 61, 62, 63, 67
Buber, Martin, 16, 24

Caring, 182
Case histories (dialogues): Bart, 130–132; David, 117, 123; Edward, 57–63; Francis, 34–39; Gilbert, 46–52; Gregory, 171–182; Jeanne, 29–33; Jonathan, 150–157; Mildred, 72–78; Will, 98–100
Catatonic phenomena, 16–17, 89
Catharsis, 46
Cézanne, Paul, 97, 139
Charcot, Jean-Martin, 14–15
Charisma, 86–87
Chesterfield, Lord, 116
Childhood, events of, and psychoses, 73
Christ, exploitation of, 39
Clearing the clinical field, 88–94
Client-centered therapy, 17
Closeness, definition of, 23

Cognition, contamination of, 89, 90, 132
Cognitive therapy, 126
Comic behavior, for shaking assumptions, 111
Commendation, 116, 147
Conditioning processes, 88
Conflict: approximating elements of, 71, 73; and bridging statements, 63; and disassociated behavior, 58; empathy of, 56–57; in "imprisoned" people, 59; intrapsychic, 161
Confrontations, 136
Confusion, patient's, 120
Contempt, 114, 115
Contradiction, of medium and message, 129–130, 132
Counterassumptive statements: definition of, 111; moving the observer, 117–123; shaking assumptions, 113–117; signaling attitudes, 112–113
Counterprojection: example of, 131; in therapy, 138–139
Counterprojective statements, 177; attack on projection, 132–137; devices for, 126–129; empathy of, 137; example of, 172; function of, 126; gaining perspective, 137–139; objections to use of, 135; resentment of, 159; uniting medium and message, 129–132
Countertransference, 92
Creativity, 93
Critic, internal, 160–162, 174
Cult leaders, 119
Cummings, E. E., 23
Cure through love, 12, 163

Darwin, Charles, 42, 43
Deflection, 128
Democratization, and projective statements, 107–109
Denial, vs. repression, 55
Depression: concept of time in, 21, 24; and counterprojection, 134; empathic statements in, 64–65; in empathic therapy, 18; existential psychiatry of, 161; and internal critic, 160–161; internalizing process

associated with, 71; phases of, 171–182; and self-depreciation, 161; and social psychiatry, 160; unloveable, 162–163; and working distance, 84
Detail, vs. abstraction, 100–102
Diagnosing process, 147
Disconfirming response, 115
Disconnection, sense of, 71
Disobedience, 15
Dissociated behavior, 58
Distance: inner, and symptomatic experience, 138; patient-analyst, 94–96; personal, management of, 83; subject-object, 68. *See also* Working distance
Domination, 4, 5, 83, 181
Doubling, 27
Doubt, 86–87

Ego, concept of, 164
Ego ideal, 148, 149, 150, 163, 167
Einstein, Albert, 24
Emotional dialectic, 49
Empathic language, 171; extensions, 67–79; finding the other, 11–25; imitative statements, 27–39
Empathic statements, 29; bridging depression and hypomania, 64–65; complex, 53–56; counterprojective force of, 133–134; example of, 155; impersonal and rhetorical or expressive, 46–52
Empathy: active vs. passive, 16–17, 43, 48, 69; affective, 19; cognitive, 19, 27; motor, 18–19; perceptual, 19; tests of, 18–20; and working distance, 85
Evolutionary theory, 93
Example, setting an, 105–107
Excitement, transmission of, 18
Exclamations, 41–43
Executive function, Freud's, 164
Existential method: and analyst-patient empathy, 6; depression vs. melancholy, 161; as feeling, 7; openness in, 90; and rhetoric, 6
Expectations, patient's, 131–132; contempt and, 115; and counterassumptive statements, 111; managing wounded, 150–157

Expressiveness, vs. manipulation, 116
Extensions: approximating elements of conflict, 71; causal, 78–79; as empathic explorations, 67–69; locating, 70–71; as "sounding the limits," 67–69; and suicidal intent, 67–69; in time and space, 67–69
Externalization, 135, 136

Facial expression, 42
Families, and psychoses, 73
Family therapy, 127–128
Fantasy, and reality, 126–127
Field. *See* Clearing the clinical field
Folie à deux, 14
Fossil diagnosis, 17
Franklin, Ben, 114
Free association, 3, 6, 91–92, 104
Freedom, concept of, 29
Freud, Sigmund, 4, 7, 12, 22, 55, 59, 88, 92, 100, 108–109, 135, 160, 163, 164

Garfield, David, 127
Gesture, 90
"God knows," 62
Goodness, and melancholic, 161
Grant, Ulysses S., 101
Group signs, 17
Group therapy, 127

Hallucinations, 137
Hardy, Thomas, 103–104
Hate, 174–178
Hazlitt, William, 116
Hendrick, Ives, 4, 18
Historical review, 60, 61
History taking, 5
"Holding open," 119
Homosexual panic, 149
Hope, 147
Hostility, 159, 172
Hypomanic character, 63–65
Hypothetical, the, 102–106, 147

Ideals, 162–164, 178–181
Identification, 160
Imagination, 24
"Imagining the real," 24
Imitative statements, 27, 28

Imperatives, 143
Impersonal, definition of, 45
"Imprisoned" person: as lacking "governance," 59; as problem of acknowledgment, 59, 63; as self-instigated, 59, 60; tools of, 60; and wish to escape, 60–62
Integration, of psychic parts, 72
"Internal damage," 154
Interpersonal language, 171; counterassumptive statements, 111–123; counterprojective statements, 125–139; and management of distance, 83–85; as managing, 7
Intimacy, and voracity, 38
Invasiveness, 84
Isolation, 4, 5, 83
Isolation of affect, as patient's defense, 51

Janet, Pierre, 7, 15
Jesenska-Pollak, Milena, 34

Kafka, Franz, 34
Kagemusha, 15–16, 25
Kernberg, Otto, 128, 138
Kleinian system, 135–136
Kohut, Heinz, 138, 167
Kraepelin, Emil, 7, 13

Languages, psychotherapeutic. *See* Empathic; Interpersonal; Performative; Projective
Leadership, charismatic, 87
"Learning perspective," 139
Le Carré, John, 113
Limit setting, 106
Lincoln, Abraham, 103
Love: cure through, 12, 163; need for, 163, 166–167, 174–178; in therapeutic relationship, 134–135

MacArthur, General Douglas, 86
Machiavelli, Nicolò, 39
Management, interpersonal, 7, 96
Manic patients, 18
Manipulation, vs. expressiveness, 116
Margulies, Alfred, 89
"Marks and remarks," 97, 126
Marx, Karl, 39

Matisse, Henri, 19
Maxim, counterassumptive statement as, 113
May, Rollo, 19–20
Medical procedures, 7, 144–146
Medium, uniting message and, 129–132
Megalomania, diagnosis of, 151, 162–163, 167
Melancholic, existential view of, 161
Mental illness, and shame, 79
Mesmer, Friedrich Anton, 15
Miller, John W., 164
Minkowski, Eugene, 21
Modesty, 103, 116, 122
Motionlessness, 21–22
Mourning, 161
Movement, dependence of psychotherapy on, 101–102

"Naked": concept of, 34; therapeutic approach to, 35–39
Napoleon, 101
Narcissism, 12, 95, 137–138, 151
Negative, in interpersonal functioning, 54–55
Neuroses, narcissistic, 12
Nietzsche, Friedrich, 39, 161
Nonverbal utterances, 42
Novey, Samuel, 139
"No wonder," 56

Obedience, 15, 85
Objective-descriptive psychiatry, 5
Observer, moving the, 117–123
Overdiagnosis, 90

"Paradoxical intention," 128
Paranoiacs, 18, 134, 136, 159
Past, and gaining perspective, 139
Pathology, loci of, 136
Perceptions, changing, and evaluation of, 19, 20
Perfectionist ideal, 148
Performative language, 147–150, 171, 179; defending self, 159–167; examples of, 144, 155, 156, 180; explained, 143; failure of, 145–147; idea of completeness or incompleteness of, 146; ideals and self, 143–

157; and internal critic, 161; and need for love, 166; negative, 165; power of, 162, 165; and self-criticism, 149
Perls, Fritz, 127
Perspective, gaining, 137–139
Play objects, 126
Poetic language, 101
Poetry, and detail, 101
Pomposity, 118, 119, 120, 122
Possession, 28, 29
Possibilities, discourse by, 93
Power: attributed to therapist, 129; balancing, 85–88; and charisma, 86; and therapeutic relationship, 88, 89
Praecoxgefuhl, 17
Praise, expectation of, 116
Predation, 11–13, 88, 89
Prisoner, patient as, 39, 59
Projection, 132, 135
Projective statements: analogy to chest percussion, 98; analogy to painting, 97; and attention, 125; counterprojective power of, 125; definition of, 97; democratizing power of, 107–109; and the hypothetical, 102–105; and the power of detail, 100–102; purpose of, 147; setting an example, 105–107; as fact or possiblity, 97; and therapist's fallibility, 108
Pronouns, 69
Proust, Marcel, 101
Proverb, counterassumptive statement as, 113
Psychoanalysis: analyst-patient alliance in, 6; and attention, 90, 92; free association in, 5–6; orthodox, 135; and self-depreciation, 161; use of imperatives in, 6
Psychodrama, 127
Psychological examination, 5
Psychosis, 60, 73, 132–134, 137

Questions, 107–108

Rage, 134–136, 182
Random, the, 22–23, 91–93
Reality and fantasy, 126–127
Reckonings, 147
Reconciliation, of psychic parts, 72

Reduction, psychological-phenomeno-
logical, 19, 90
Reich, Wilhelm, 7
Repression, vs. denial, 55
Resistances, 47
Respect, 88, 107
Responsibility, 39
Rhetoric, 45–46
Rogers, Carl, 17, 45
Rorschach test, 93, 94, 127

Sarton, May, 122
Schizophrenia, 13, 22, 24, 71, 90
Self: defending, 143, 159–167; and
ideals, 162–164; and need for love,
164; search for, 120; transformation
of, 167
Self-criticism, 115, 148–149, 161, 173,
177
Self-deception, 59
Self-esteem, 154, 160, 164
Self-possession, concept of, 28
Self-watchfulness, development of, 13
Semrad, Elvin, 5, 70
Shrewdness, in psychopathic charisma,
86–87
Simulation, 37
Size, experience of, 23
Skepticism, vs. contempt, 114
Slavery, 88, 89
Social training, of men vs. women, 112
Space: disorders of, 22–23; and em-
pathic therapy, 96; and extensions,
67–69, 70–72; and finding the
other, 21–25; psychopathology of,
22
Strachey, Lytton, 103–104
Subject-object differentiation, 5, 6
Submission, 4, 5, 13
Suicidal intent, and extensions, 67–68
Sullivan, Harry Stack, 5, 6, 18, 42, 57,
62, 90, 139

Superego, 148, 149, 150, 162–164
Supine patients, explained, 3, 161
Surprise, and empathic stance, 44

Talion principle, 109
Thanatos, 136
Thematic Apperception Test, 127
Therapists: authority of, 165; charac-
teristics of, 135, 146; and integrated
psychotherapy, 7–8; and passion,
182
"Thrown," 22, 23
Thurber, James, 121
Time: contrasts real and perceived, 68;
disorders of, 21, 22; and extensions,
67–69, 70–72; and finding the
other, 21–25
Tolerance, 96
Transference, 106, 108, 127–128,
132–134, 138, 167
Translations, 42–45, 67, 73
Truth, and the hypothetical, 104

Uncertainty, 31, 121
Unexpectedness, 22

Validation, as function of empathic
translations, 45, 51
Values, *See* Ideals
Verdictives, explained, 147

Warfare, and detail, 101
Will, 86–87
Winnicott, D. W., 7, 84, 126
Wishes, vs. "audience," 152
Wishing for, as performative, 147
Women, social training of, 112
"Wonder," 55–56, 64
Working alliance, 134
Working distance, 88, 143; and being
alone together, 84–85; and empathy,
85; between patient and therapist,
36–39, 84–85